DSM-IV DIAGNOSIS IN THE SCHOOLS

The Guilford School Practitioner Series

EDITORS

STEPHEN N. ELLIOTT, PhD
Univeristy of Wisconsin–Madison

JOSEPH C. WITT, PhD
Louisiana State University, Baton Rouge

Recent Volumes

Assessment for Early Intervention: Best Practices for Professionals
STEPHEN J. BAGNATO and JOHN T. NEISWORTH

The Clinical Child Interview
JAN N. HUGHES and DAVID B. BAKER

Working with Families in Crisis: School-Based Intervention
WILLIAM STEELE and MELVYN RAIDER

Practitioner's Guide to Dynamic Assessment
CAROL S. LIDZ

Reading Problems: Consultation and Remediation
P. G. AARON and R. MALATESHA JOSHI

Crisis Intervention in the Schools
GAYLE D. PITCHER and SCOTT POLAND

Behavior Change in the Classroom: Self-Management Interventions
EDWARD S. SHAPIRO and CHRISTINE L. COLE

ADHD in the Schools: Assessment and Intervention Strategies
GEORGE J. DuPAUL and GARY STONER

School Interventions for Children of Alcoholics
BONNIE K. NASTASI and DENISE M. DeZOLT

Entry Strategies for School Consultation
EDWARD S. MARKS

Instructional Consultation Teams: Collaborating for Change
SYLVIA A. ROSENFIELD and TODD A. GRAVOIS

Social Problem Solving: Interventions in the Schools
MAURICE J. ELIAS and STEVEN E. TOBIAS

Academic Skills Problems: Direct Assessment and Intervention, Second Edition
EDWARD S. SHAPIRO

Brief Intervention for School Problems: Collaborating for Practical Solutions
JOHN J. MURPHY and BARRY L. DUNCAN

Advanced Applications of Curriculum-Based Measurement
MARK R. SHINN, Editor

Medications for School-Age Children: Effects on Learning and Behavior
RONALD T. BROWN and MICHAEL G. SAWYER

DSM-IV Diagnosis in the Schools
ALVIN E. HOUSE

DSM-IV Diagnosis in the Schools

♦♦♦

Alvin E. House

♦

THE GUILFORD PRESS
New York   London

©1999; revisions ©2002 The Guilford Press
A Division of Guilford Publications, Inc.
72 Spring Street, New York, NY 10012
www.guilford.com

Printed in the United States of America

This book is printed on acid-free paper.

Last digit is print number: 9 8 7 6 5 4

Library of Congress Cataloging-in-Publication Data

House, Alvin E.
 DSM-IV diagnosis in the schools / Alvin E. House.
  p. cm. — (The Guilford school practitioner series)
 Includes bibliographical references and index.
 ISBN 1-57230-759-5
 1. Mental illness—Diagnosis. 2. Child psychopathology.
3. School children—Mental health. I. Series. II. Title.
III. Series.
RJ503.5.H68 1999
618.92′890075—DC21   98-19601
                          CIP

About the Author

♦

Alvin E. House is a clinical psychologist whose professional practice focuses on applying assessment results in school, vocational, medical, and forensic consultations. As Associate Professor in the Psychology Department at Illinois State University, Normal, he routinely teaches graduate level courses in mental health diagnosis, psychological assessment, and psychopathology. He has coauthored a manual on observational assessment of children as well as journal articles and book chapters on intellectual, personality, and neuropsychological testing.

Acknowledgments

♦

I would like to express my appreciation for the support and encouragement of my wife, Betty House, and our children, Tiechera and Brannan. They put up with long periods of unavailability as I tried to create meaning on a monitor screen. I would also like to thank my colleague Larry Alferink, who as chair of the Department of Psychology at Illinois State University did his best to sustain an environment in which teaching and scholarly work could be conducted. Finally, I would like to applaud the faith and persistence of my editor at The Guilford Press, Sharon Panulla, who believed in this project and worked for its realization.

Contents

◆

Introduction:
Purposes and Features
of This Book

◆

WHAT THIS BOOK IS—AND IS NOT—INTENDED TO DO

Efficient and accurate use of the American Psychiatric Association's (1994a) *Diagnostic and Statistical Manual of Mental Disorders,* fourth edition (DSM-IV) has become a necessary part of the professional duties of psychologists in a variety of clinical, rehabilitative, and child service agencies. For several reasons this development has extended into public school systems, where school psychologists are increasingly being asked to make DSM-IV diagnostic determinations. Doll's (1996) review of epidemiological studies concluded that "a typical school of 1,000 students could be expected to have between 180 and 220 students with diagnosable psychiatric disorders" (p. 29). This book is intended to increase child psychologists' familiarity with DSM-IV and to bolster their confidence in using it within school settings. The use of DSM-IV is often made difficult by both the size of the text (886 pages) and the complexity of the taxonomy (approximately 320 diagnoses). Some of the rules and conventions adopted to bring increased structure and reliability to the system add further to the complexity of the document for novice users. These considerations, combined with timidity about using a "medical" system, may leave neophytes feeling totally confused and frustrated. The present text attempts to provide a broad understanding of the DSM-IV system—what it attempts to do, how it is organized, and how to use it most effectively to

1

capture and communicate the unique features of children's and adolescent's problems.

The present book does *not* take the place of DSM-IV. Any psychologist who plans to use DSM-IV will need a copy of it (see the Professional Note). Several fine books are available on using DSM-IV; significant amounts of text in these volumes are often devoted to paraphrasing the DSM category definitions and diagnostic criteria. This adds to the size and cost of these books—but it does not eliminate the need to have a copy of DSM-IV. The present book, unlike these others, does not repeat or paraphrase DSM-IV categories. Instead, it shows how the system is organized and how this organization relates to common presenting problems, as well as to other classification systems readers may be familiar with.

Related to the issue of having a copy of DSM-IV available is the question of attempting to memorize the criteria. Various memory aids have been developed for previous diagnostic categories. Reeves and Bullen (1995) have published mnemonics for 10 of the DSM-IV Mental Disorders or syndromes: Major Depression, Mania, Dysthymia, Generalized Anxiety Disorder, Posttraumatic Stress Disorder, Panic Attack, Anorexia Nervosa, Bulimia Nervosa, Delirium, and Borderline Personality Disorder. Although there are probably useful appli-

---

**PROFESSIONAL NOTE	Best Practice Regarding the Availability of a Copy of DSM-IV**

I would advise psychologists to have a copy of DSM-IV itself available in every setting they practice in. This diagnostic system cannot be used reliably or accurately without access to the diagnostic criteria and associated features for the categories. The *Quick Reference to the Diagnostic Criteria from DSM-IV* (American Psychiatric Association, 1994b) can be a useful reference in certain situations. This small book contains only the diagnostic criteria and IDC-9-CM numerical codes for the DSM-IV diagnoses; it is portable and easy to skim over, even within an evaluation session. But the *Quick Reference* omits both the text discussions and the associated features for the diagnoses. In many diagnostic decisions, especially the difficult ones, a careful consideration of the features commonly associated with various categories is essential in determining the most parsimonious but complete classification. This information must be available to examiners if their diagnostic decisions are to be informed ones. A copy of DSM-IV should be readily available in each setting where diagnoses are formulated.

---

cations for such devices, in general I do not advise attempting to memorize diagnostic categories. There are several reason for this, but a strong pragmatic one is the sheer number of categories and criteria in DSM-IV. It is probably far more efficient to use the *Quick Reference* (American Psychiatric Association, 1994b) as a prompt or to develop one's own checklist than to try to learn dozens of mnemonics for even the most common disorders seen in children. Having a general idea of the overall structure of DSM-IV is very helpful, but I believe that memorizing lists is of very limited usefulness to the professional psychologist.

A GUIDE TO STYLISTIC CONVENTIONS IN THIS BOOK

One feature of DSM-IV that contributes slightly to its length but significantly to its lack of accessibility to many readers is the decision of its authors not to use acronyms, even very commonly employed ones. For example, "Attention-Deficit/Hyperactivity Disorder" and "Posttraumatic Stress Disorder" are used throughout the text, whereas many publications would use these full phrases once and thereafter refer to "ADHD" and "PSTD." There are both advantages and disadvantages to this decision. The authors of DSM-IV have striven for a clarity and specificity of communication often absent from diagnostic writings. They try to say exactly what they mean, using full details rather than expecting the reader to infer what is meant. Although "ADHD" is a commonly used expression in the mental health literature, and is probably familiar to almost any potential user of DSM-IV, "ADHD" in the literature does not always mean the same as "Attention-Deficit/Hyperactivity Disorder" as defined within DSM-IV. By stating explicitly what they mean, the authors prevent possible misunderstanding or misinterpretation. They will on occasion use an acronym for one of their own expressions (e.g., "NOS" for "Not Otherwise Specified"), but even this convention is very limited. The avoidance of acronyms can be an advantage for the occasional user of DSM-IV, who does not need to refer constantly to a key to decipher terms found in the text: "Now what did that mean?" The cost of this clarity, however, is a rather ponderous text, and the occasional reader can sometimes become lost in the prose.

In the present book, several common acronyms are used for the sake of brevity. When the name of a diagnostic entity is first used in a chapter, the full term is provided and the acronym to be used subsequently is then given in parentheses: for example, "Attention-Deficit/Hyperactivity Disorder (ADHD)." These acronyms are used within this text to stand for the entities as defined within the DSM system.

A second stylistic convention used in this book pertains to diagnostic entities from the various editions of DSM. Diagnostic categories from DSM-IV are given in the text with the first letter of each word capitalized, but without further elaboration: for example, "Conduct Disorder." Diagnostic categories from previous editions of DSM are always identified according to the edition they came from: for example, "Conduct Disorder (DSM-III)" or "in DSM-III, Conduct Disorder . . . ." The exact definitions of Conduct Disorder and most other categories have changed across the different editions of DSM. Many of these changes are subtle and possibly have had little effect on use or results. Some changes, however, have had significant effects on the populations identified with the revised categories (Volkmar, Bregman, Cohen, & Cicchetti, 1988). Unfortunately, we often cannot know what the impact of specific wording or criterion changes have been until we are informed by subsequent research. Clearly, it appears not to be a good idea to assume much about the effects of changes in wording, symptom criteria, or frequency criteria on the application of a diagnostic category. Given this, within the present discussion "Conduct Disorder" or its acronym, "CD," means the category as defined within DSM-IV; "Conduct Disorder (DSM-III)" or CD (DSM-III)" means the category as defined within DSM-III; and "conduct disorder" or "conduct problem" has the general meaning that would be assigned to it in the psychological literature.

A third convention used herein pertains to references. References to any source other than DSM-IV (including previous versions of DSM) follow the usual style of the American Psychological Association: author, year, and page number if relevant. In references to the text of DSM-IV, only a page number will be given. All page-number-only references should be assumed to refer to the full text version of DSM-IV (American Psychiatric Association, 1994a).

THE FOUR TYPES OF NOTES AND THEIR PURPOSES

I have used four different types of notes as "sidebars" in this book to draw certain issues to the reader's attention. "Coding Notes" pertain to the use of the DSM-IV diagnostic system to classify the problems of children and adolescents. Some Coding Notes identify common errors in practice so that these can be avoided; others indicate changes in the ICD-9-CM (*International Classification of Diseases*, 9th revision, Clinical Modification [ICD-9-CM; World Health Organization, 1991]) numerical codes for several DSM-IV categories; and still others present supplemental material not directly pertaining to DSM-IV, but relevant to the broader activity of psychodiagnosis.

"Application Notes" have to do with "decoding" the diagnoses given by other professionals, and understanding as fully as possible the information being presented. Application Notes attempt to clarify not only the formal conventions of DSM-IV, but also common practices in medical reports and other professional communications. A psychiatric diagnosis is always a summary description for an extremely complex phenomenon—the actions of another human being. In any classification effort, a certain amount of idiosyncratic information is sacrificed in order to gain the usefulness of nomothetic similarities. The challenge for the examiner is to capture the most valuable (informative) feature of a child's or adolescents' presentation in the diagnoses used. The challenge for the reader is to understand as fully as possible what information is being offered by other practitioners. Application Notes will attempt to aid this understanding.

"Professional Notes" (such as the Professional Note on p. 2) identify "best-practice recommendations"—suggestions about diagnostic practice that are aimed at ensuring the highest level of professional psychological care for clients. Working to ensure the best service to clients, employers, and colleagues gives practicing psychologists both their best protection from personal liability and their greatest reward in personal satisfaction and professional pride. Professional Notes attempt to identify both essential elements of competent practices and exemplary levels of professional care.

Finally, "IDEA Notes" comment on the potential relationships between DSM-IV diagnoses and classifications of eligibility for special services under the Individuals with Disabilities Education Act (IDEA; Public Law 101-476) and its amendments. Services to children are provided within the context of a number of conceptual and classification systems. Understanding the interrelationship between DSM-IV and other frameworks of understanding—in this case, that of the U.S. government—can greatly enhance the utility of mental health diagnosis for practicing school and child clinical psychologists.

2002 UPDATES: IDEA 1997 AND DSM-IV-TR

Although the essential features of DSM-IV have remained the same across the first 7 years of its use, there have been a number of changes. The ICD-9-CM numerical codes, for instance, have undergone some minor revisions. When DSM-IV was published in 1994, there was one

ICD-9-CM code for Conduct Disorder, regardless of subtype: 312.8. The two subtypes, based on age of onset, were noted in the DSM-IV diagnosis but were not represented in the World Health Organization classification coding. This was changed in 1996 to decimalized codes for the subtypes: 312.81 for Childhood-Onset Type, 312.82 for Adolescent-Onset Type, and 312.89 for Unspecified Onset (see the Coding Note on p. 49). Even the published edition of a book is not a completely static entry.

Two important events pertaining to the topic of this text that have occurred since its initial appearance in 1999 were the publication of the final regulations applying the 1997 Amendments to the Individuals with Disabilities Education Act (IDEA 1997; Public Law 105-17) in the *Federal Register* on March 12, 1999, and the publication in 2000 of the text revision to the fourth edition of the *Diagnostic and Statistical Manual of Mental Disorders* (DSM-IV-TR; American Psychiatric Association, 2000). One feature of this book is pointing out the points of intersection and divergence between the categories of qualification for special education services under IDEA and the diagnostic entries of DSM. The appearance of IDEA 1997 shifts somewhat this relationship. A more dramatic event was the publication of a revision of the DSM manual itself. Since the central purpose of this book is to help readers appreciate the application of the DSM system to youth, it is certainly reasonable to question how this application has been affected by the changes embodied in DSM-IV-TR. As it turns out, like the subtle elaboration of the ICD codes, the overall impact of these two events on the use of DSM-IV is not great. To make readers aware of the changes, a limited amount of additional material has been added to the fourth printing of this book (see new text and IDEA and Coding Notes beginning on p. 231).

PART I

♦♦♦

DIAGNOSTIC ISSUES
AND THE USE OF DSM-IV

♦

The initial task in learning to use DSM-IV is understanding what is involved in a mental health diagnosis. The general issues involved in psychiatric classification and the specific ways of operationalizing these issues developed by the authors of DSM-IV shape much of DSM-IV's resulting taxonomy. School and child psychologists usually have a general sense of the "medical model" derived from their graduate couses in abnormal behavior or developmental psychopathology, but the perspectives of DSM-IV reflects the efforts of almost a century of articulating a particular view for understanding human problems. In this perspective the clinician assumes a pivotal role. Chapter 1 explores this underlying model of the diagnostic process and the professional examiner's crucial contribution to and responsibility in applying it. Chapter 2 provides an overview of the DSM clssification model and the important constructs used within this system. Chapter 3 addresses the process of learning to use DSM-IV.

CHAPTER 1

♦♦♦

Psychiatric Diagnosis:
Issues for School Psychologists

♦

THE EMERGENCE OF PSYCHIATRIC DIAGNOSIS
AS A TASK IN SCHOOL SETTINGS

Traditional educational and psychological assessment within school settings began with psychometric measurement of cognitive abilities and academic achievement, and evolved to include evaluations of behavioral adjustment and personality. The results of these evaluations were usually communicated in descriptive narratives, with or without accompanying standard scores. Diagnostic classification was typically limited to a statement of eligibility for services (e.g., "eligible for special education") and perhaps a broad designation of the area of eligibility (e.g., "behavior-disordered"). Although most school psychologists were probably aware, on a professional level, of the publication of the landmark third edition of DSM (DSM-III; American Psychiatric Association, 1980), it had little direct impact on their practice or daily work activities. By the time DSM-III-R was published (American Psychiatric Association, 1987), the situation had begun to change, and publications and workshops addressing the use of DSM in school settings began to appear. The publication of DSM-IV in 1994 occurred in the context of broad economic, political, and social changes in the delivery of mental health services in the United States. These changes have, among many other effects, brought psychiatric diagnosis within the assigned tasks of an increasing number of school psychologists.

The current forces driving the increased interest in formal medical diagnosis of children's behavior and learning problems reflect the changing economic realities affecting many school districts. Despite occasional denouncements of school districts' "extravagance," the continued enactment of mandated services without accompanying mandated funding has increased the financial burden on many schools. Coincident with this has been the increased difficulty in obtaining school funding from traditional tax sources. The search for alternative funding sources to help relieve the expense of mandated programs has led to an interest in tapping into third-party reimbursement (i.e., commercial and governmental health insurance) for psychological services provided within schools.

It is at this point that DSM enters the picture, because, among the other roles played by psychiatric diagnosis, it clearly serves the primary "gatekeeping" function for insurance companies and government agencies in determining reimbursement decisions. If the school district is to gain access to potential sources of mental health service reimbursement, it is necessary for a qualified professional to determine appropriate DSM-IV classifications and corresponding ICD-9-CM numerical codes for insurance review consideration. Thus psychiatric diagnosis has increasingly become part of the task of school psychologists. The expanded attention given to diagnostic classification can be seen in the recent miniseries devoted to the topic in *School Psychology Review* (Power & DuPaul, 1996a).

PSYCHIATRIC CLASSIFICATION
AND ITS ROLE IN SCHOOL SETTINGS

Psychological assessment is a broad process that encompasses many different approaches to understanding and measuring human actions and adjustment. The activities usually involved in mental health assessment differ in some important ways from the evaluation procedures traditionally used by school psychologists. First, DSM represents a categorical classification system; that is, the goal in using it is to arrive at a category or categories that most accurately reflect a child's adjustment and functioning at this time. The purposes served by classification can include the assignment of treatment or other appropriate disposition; efficient communication with other professionals; and statistical record keeping for use in program planning, outcome research, or other application.

In addition, this classification process depends crucially upon the clinical judgment and decision making of the individual mental health professional. Psychologists need to keep in mind that DSM-IV is a document written primarily by physicians and intended primarily for the use of physicians. The working perspective in medicine is that of an individual practitioner who actively assembles relevant data, evaluates the data, arrives at working diagnoses, and acts upon the diagnoses to provide appropriate interventions. The considerable degree of authority and responsibility that the practitioner thus assumes is somewhat foreign to the practice traditions of many allied health professions. Psychology has evolved out of an academic tradition that values careful development of positions, cautious formulations of hypotheses, and consensual decisions. When I was a clinical psychology intern in a medical center, a psychiatrist on staff who supervised me pointed out to me a difference he had observed in the typical oral presentations of psychology interns and psychiatry residents. The interns tended to communicate by carefully stating all the data and the rationales leading up to their final diagnostic conclusions, whereas the residents had learned to begin by stating their diagnostic impressions and, if there were questions, following these assertions up with their observations and rationales. This proved to be a very valuable lesson for me—both in dealing with physicians, but in beginning to understand the consequences of differences in professional training and traditions. In using DSM-IV, it is helpful to recognize that the judgment and decision of the professional practitioner usually serve as the basis for classification.

Although there are significant issues to be considered regarding the use of categorical diagnostic classifications with clients, especially with children, most of these are not addressed in detail here. Even to sketch the outlines of this topic would exceed the desired length of this text. Waldman and Lilienfeld (1995) present a good discussion of many of the issues involved in the diagnosis and classification of psychiatric syndromes in children. Critiques of the DSM approach in general (Kirk & Kutchins, 1992) and of DSM-IV in particular (Blashfield & Fuller, 1996; Kutchins & Kirk, 1995) have appeared, and others will follow. This is desirable for the positive evolution of our efforts to understand and classify childhood behavior problems.

For the purposes of the present book, however, it is assumed that a decision to use psychiatric diagnoses for classification purposes has already been made. Given this decision, the question becomes this: How can the DSM classification system be used to yield the most reliable, accurate, and useful results? This text is intended to help the reader become familiar with the main features of this approach to understanding and classifying emotional, behavioral, and cognitive disturbances in adjustment. In particular, I have tried to help bridge the differences in orientation and training between the school psychologists who are increasingly being called upon to use this classification system in their work setting, and the practicing physicians for whom DSM was primarily intended.

DEVELOPMENTAL FEATURES TO CONSIDER IN DIAGNOSING CHILDREN AND ADOLESCENTS

Although, as I have stated above, space considerations preclude a detailed debate of the merits and demerits of a categorical diagnostic system such as DSM-IV, most commentators agree that the application of such a system to children and adolescents is especially challenging. In this section, I discuss some of the developmental features that must be taken into consideration in the psychiatric diagnosis of children and adolescents.

A typical adult client presents himself or herself to a mental health professional and reports the concerns that have led him or her to seek services—for instance, sadness and crying spells, discouraging marital conflicts, or questions about career direction. The most commonly utilized assessment tool/approach is the clinical interview. Based upon the verbal information reported by the adult client, the professional arrives at an assessment (which may include a DSM diagnosis), proposes a treatment plan, and makes a disposition of the case. Often implicit in this exchange are the assumptions that the client's report of his or her circumstances are largely accurate; that the client's personality and cognitive functioning are relatively stable over time; and that (within certain ethical boundaries) the agenda of therapy is largely shaped by the client's wishes and goals. These modal features of work with adults influence many aspects of caregiving, including the practices leading to diagnosis.

Professionals working primarily with children and adolescents deal routinely with very different initial characteristics. Young persons almost never refer themselves for treatment or other psychological services; they are referred by adult caretakers (parents, teachers, other concerned adults) who have become concerned about their adjustment, functioning, progress, or happiness. A basic truism is that the things children and adolescents may worry about most may not be the things that concern their caretakers most. For instance, fears of animals are the most common extreme anxiety reactions of children, fears of animals are not the most commonly seen fears in professional practice with children. Fears of school are not frequent among children's anxiety problems; however, school phobia is one of the most commonly seen and investigated childhood fears in clinical circumstances (Miller, Barrett, & Hampe, 1974). This disparity illustrates one of the most important factors in assessing child and adolescent psychopathology: young children are referred by adults because of behavior that causes the adults concern. This has profound implications for what problems are noticed, are studied, become better understood, and evolve into recognized diagnostic entries.

Children and adolescents also appear to be more influenced by environmental variables than adults; their behavior is more situationally specific. Many aspects of young persons' adjustment and functioning, including their problems, are more fluid and evolving than is the case for most adults. This creates problems for categorical classification systems, in which it is assumed that the classified things or individuals remain relatively constant unless they are deliberately changed. This greater responsiveness to environmental contingencies also means that a greater degree of attention must be devoted to evaluating situational characteristics and variables in arriving at an understanding or diagnosis of young people's problems. For instance, the change in DSM-IV from basing a diagnosis of Attention-Deficit/ Hyperactivity Disorder (ADHD) upon symptoms in only one setting to requiring manifestation of symptoms in at least two settings greatly affects the identified population and its modal characteristics. Requiring cross-situational manifestation (pervasive ADHD) reduces the number of children identified as having ADHD, may reduce false-positive diagnoses, may increase false-negative diagnoses, and probably leads to a focus on more severely disturbed children—thereby altering the modal features of a child diagnosed with ADHD.

In addition to the need to attend to environmental features, the language and cognitive differences between youth and adults must be taken into consideration. A primary reliance on verbal reports in the context of a clinical interview is often seen as a much less acceptable data base for evaluating children and adolescents than for evaluating adults. For example, clinically depressed children, especially preschool and early primary school children, may not report themselves to be sad. They may report physical concerns or vague complaints of "not feeling well." Their nonverbal behavior may prompt others to express concerns about their well-being. They may show, but not necessarily report, a decrease in activities they previously enjoyed. In the words of one of my students, children tend to "walk the walk" of depression rather than "talk the talk." Interviews with parents and other collateral informants, behavior rating scales, naturalistic observations, and formal psychological testing all play a relatively more important role in the assessment of children and adolescents than in that of adults. These differences have implications for the use of DSM-IV with children and adolescents, and bring into focus some of the recurrent dissatisfactions with the DSM system. In this book, I try to point out occasions in which additional sources of information can be especially useful in applying DSM-IV classifications to the evaluation of young people.

CHAPTER 2

◆◆◆

An Overview of the DSM-IV Diagnostic System

◆

BASIC DEFINITIONS OF MENTAL DISORDERS AND OTHER CONDITIONS

DSM-IV is concerned with classifying mental disorders. There are several things to take into account in order to understand exactly what is meant by this statement. One is the meaning of "mental disorder"— that is, the criteria by which a decision is made that a mental disorder exists. One also must take into account the relationship between mental disorders and other phenomena of interest—especially the observable characteristics of individuals, their self-reports, and theories of the cause and prevention of mental disorders.

DSM-IV offers a definition of "Mental Disorder," as did DSM-III and DSM-III-R. There are only minor differences among these. Since DSM-III, the cognitive and behavioral disorders classified by DSM-IV as Mental Disorders have been identified by means of one or both of two defining characteristics: significant personal distress in the individual affected and/or significant adaptive failure. The additional criteria discussed can be viewed as various special cases of the second criterion. Each and every time the term "disorder" is used in DSM-IV in the context of a mental, emotional, or behavioral problem, the meaning is that in addition to any other specific criteria that are met, one or both of these two general criteria are also met. All Mental Disorders, by definition, meet this basic criterion:

> In DSM-IV, each of the mental disorders is conceptualized as a clinically significant behavioral or psychological syndrome or pattern that occurs in an individual and that is associated with present distress (e.g.,

a painful symptom) or disability (i.e., impairment in one or more important areas of functioning) or with a significantly increased risk of suffering death, pain, disability, or an important loss of freedom. (DSM-IV, 1994a, p. xxi)

The discussion in the text goes on to exclude expectable responses to a particular event (such as the death of a loved one); to require that the problem currently be considered a behavioral, psychological, or biological dysfunction in the person (regardless of what its original cause may have been); and to address the boundaries of social deviance and mental disorder: "Neither deviant behavior (e.g., political, religious, or sexual) nor conflicts that are primarily between the individual and society are mental disorders unless the deviance or conflict is a symptom of a dysfunction in the individual, as described above" (p. xxii). A very important feature of the DSM system has been the formal declaration (since DSM-III) that the classification is not a classification of people, but rather of the disorders that people experience.

The idea of a disorder, mental or otherwise, involves a perception of an enduring group of associated characteristics. The basic elements are objective data about an individual and his or her (subjective) self-reports. A "sign" is some observable (measurable), objective characteristic of the person. For example, increased heart rate, perspiration, and behavioral avoidance when confronted with a feared object would be several signs of anxiety in a client. A "symptom" refers to the subjective report of the person. The client's statements that he or she is fearful, is nervous, and wishes to get away from the feared situation are all symptoms of anxiety. The observation or statistical determination that a number of signs and symptoms may go together forms the basis of identification of syndromes. "Syndromes" are patterns of covariation between signs and symptoms. There is a trend toward increased consistency among authors in their use of these three terms. Signs, symptoms, and syndromes provide the basic elements of many modern conceptualizations of emotional and behavior problems, including the DSM.

The Criterion A requirements of most of the DSM-IV diagnoses identify the relevant syndrome for each diagnosis. A syndrome is what many students tend to think of as the defining feature of a Mental Disorder, but there are usually other elements just as important and essential. There may also be inclusion of requirements of duration. Some syndromes are identified as an event. The discussion of "panic attack," which is used as the core element of several anxiety disorder definitions, is given as several signs and symptoms occurring together.

This is a classical presentation of a syndrome. The discussion of mood disorders illustrates the use of time requirements. A major depressive syndrome is specified with the additional requirement that the cluster of symptoms and signs have occurred for a minimum of two weeks: this is identified as a "depressive episode." There may also be exclusion criteria—identification of other problems (Mental Disorders or General Medical Conditions) which would preclude a given diagnosis being made if they were present.

A disorder is, then, identified as a syndrome that meets certain additional criteria. In DSM-IV, the requirements for all disorders are evidence of significant personal distress, functional impairment, or contribution to personal risk of loss (see the basic definition of "mental disorder," above). One change from DSM-III-R to DSM-IV has been the overt inclusion of these requirements in most of the diagnostic criterion sets. This does not represent any conceptual change—the requirement was there as early as DSM-III—but these fundamental requirements were not repeated over and over. The decision to add them (as several lines of text) to most DSM-IV criterion sets is an attempt to decrease overdiagnosis of subclinical problems by reminding examiners that all mental disorders not only must meet the specific criteria for a particular type of behavioral or emotional problem, but must also show the characteristics that define psychopathology for DSM-IV. The fundamental task of the examiner in using DSM-IV is to decide whether the human difficulties he or she is presented with can be reasonably conceptualized as mental disorders within the DSM system.

An "illness" is a disorder with known etiology and pathophysiology; that is, a full understanding exists of the causes and mechanisms of the problems. Very few of the disorders defined in DSM-IV are close to the point where they might be conceptualized as illnesses. Indeed, some would maintain that most human behavioral enactments cannot be reasonably considered as illnesses with "illness" so defined. Nevertheless, recent developments in the study of several mental disorders raise intriguing possibilities that at least a few may ultimately be understood in this form. This type of understanding is often one of the goals of medical research, and the expansion of our knowledge about behavioral and emotional problems may require a fundamental reorganization of our view of some of these problems. Some research on autism, for instance, suggests this pattern of behavior and maladjustment may be a final common pathway of several etiological processes, some of which may ultimately be well conceptualized as illnesses. These topics, however, are far beyond the scope of this book, which focuses on the application of the current DSM diagnostic system.

Mental disorders are not the only problems classified in DSM-IV. Various human relationship difficulties and other conditions that cause upset in adjustment and functioning are considered, because these problems are frequently the focus of clinical attention. These "Other Conditions That May Be a Focus of Clinical Attention" provide for the specification of a wide range of problematic circumstances in the lives of individuals being evaluated. Many of these other conditions may be among the problems most frequently seen by the practicing psychologist or counselor. These problems are viewed as important within DSM-IV, and there are provisions for coding them, but they are not mental disorders within the meaning of that term in DSM-IV. These problems are not mental disorders because they do not meet the basic requirements for a mental disorder—significant distress, functional impairment, and/or special risk. The defining aspect of these other conditions is that in the judgment of the examiner, they warrant clinical attention. An easy operationalization of this idea would be the development of a treatment plan to address one of these other conditions, or inclusion of the problem as a specific treatment target in the intervention plan for a related mental disorder. Identification of one or more other conditions in a child's or adolescent's diagnosis does not require such formal justification, but there is the clear implication that these are serious difficulties for the young person and justify some attention. They are discussed in more detail below.

The consideration that a problem is severe enough to be a focus of treatment is a general criterion used in identifying Other Conditions, as well as in deciding at the time whether to make an additional, separate diagnosis of an associated symptom area when the youth has an identified Mental Disorder. For instance, a Sleep Disorder would not normally be diagnosed in a teenager with Major Depressive Disorder because sleep problems are symptoms of depression; however, if treatment of the sleep disturbance is judged to be a critical treatment focus, an independent diagnosis can be made.

In addition to Other Conditions, various psychological, social, and medical characteristics of a child or adolescent may be classified within DSM-IV and do not constitute Mental Disorders. Before these are described, it is necessary to take a look at the overall organization of classification in DSM-IV—the multiaxial nature of the classification.

MULTIAXIAL CLASSIFICATION

Beginning with DSM-III in 1980, the American Psychiatric Association's diagnostic system was structured around five "axes" or categories of information (see the following Coding Note). Multiaxial approaches to diagnosis were recommended as a means of ensuring a more complete assessment of each client as a total person— that is, of encouraging a review of several aspects of adjustment and functioning, rather than just symptoms. Each of the two subsequent revisions of DSM have seen slight modifications of the axes' content, but the basic structure has been left intact. The term "axis" may be somewhat misleading for the reader if it is taken to imply a dimensional or continuous variable. Only one of the axes—Axis V, Global Assessment of Functioning—constitutes a continuous scale. The other axes involve various categorical classifications of different types of information: acute clinical problems, enduring characteristics of the individual, medical conditions, and environmental stressors.

Axis I: Clinical Disorders and Other Conditions
That May Be Focus of Clinical Attention

The basic body of DSM-IV is contained in the diagnoses made on Axis I. These are the acute clinical conditions that usually bring a client to an examiner's attention. Most Axis I disorders are viewed as afflictions that have developed in a client's life at some point ("onset"); trouble the client over some period of time ("course"); and,

---

CODING NOTE   The Multiaxial Classification of DSM-IV

Axis I	Clinical Disorders are coded.
	Other Conditions That May Be a Focus of Clinical Attention (often called "V codes") are coded.
Axis II	Mental Retardation is coded.
	Personality Disorders are coded.
	Also, personality traits and ego defences may be noted (though these are not coded).
Axis III	General Medical Conditions and other relevant health information are noted.
Axis IV	Psychosocial and Environmental Problems are listed.
Axis V	Global Assessment of Functioning (GAF) is rated.

---

one hopes, are resolved either in the natural course of events or through treatment ("remission"). Unless noted otherwise, the first diagnosis listed on Axis I is assumed to be the problem that brought the client to the examiner's attention (or, in the case of a child or adolescent, led a caretaker to seek clinical attention for the youngster).

Many diagnoses can be further differentiated by the use of "subtypes" and "specifiers." Subtypes are "mutually exclusive and jointly exhaustive" patterns of phenomenological characteristics (p. 1). For example, Conduct Disorder has two subtypes based on the age of onset of problems: Childhood-Onset Type and Adolescent-Onset Type. Specifiers are "not intended to be mutually exclusive or jointly exhaustive," but instead "provide an opportunity to define a more homogeneous subgrouping of individuals" within a diagnostic category (p. 1). In a diagnosis of Stereotypic Movement Disorder, for instance, a specifier is available: With Self-Injurious Behavior. The logic behind the distinction between subtypes and specifies is not always clear, and the reader will simply have to follow the directions for the particular diagnosis being considered. For example, age of onset is used as a subtyping principle for Conduct Disorder, but for Separation Anxiety Disorder a single specifier is available: Early Onset.

Severity specifiers are a frequently employed class of specifiers in DSM-IV. The specifiers Mild, Moderate, and Severe may be used when a case meets full criteria for any diagnosis; for several diagnoses, explicit criteria for the specifiers are provided. Both frequency and qualitative features are considered in choosing a severity specifier. The designation Mild is used when the manifest symptoms only just meet the diagnostic criteria requirements for the category. Severe usually means that many more symptoms than the minimum necessary for diagnosis can be documented. Moderate is used to qualify cases with an intermediate frequency of symptoms between Mild and Severe. The assignment of a severity specifier, however, is complicated by the additional consideration of the intensity and/or functional impact of symptoms.

As an illustration, consider Conduct Disorder again. This diagnosis requires the presence of at least 3 of 15 symptoms during the past year. I would usually qualify the Conduct Disorder diagnosis of a child with 3 or 4 symptoms as Mild, would use Severe for a child with 12 or more symptoms, and would use Moderate somewhere in between these extremes. But the assignment of Mild requires few symptoms in excess of the required 3 *and* only minor harm to others, whereas the assignment of Severe requires many conduct problems beyond the 3 needed for criteria or "considerable harm to others" (pp. 87, 91). A child who often bullies other children at school, initiates frequent fights on a regular basis, and has violently beaten another child with a baseball bat will probably be diagnosed as having Conduct Disorder, Severe, on the basis of the harm caused in the one attack with a weapon. My experience suggests that intra- and interrater reliability rates in the use of severity specifiers are probably significantly lower than agreement on the basic diagnosis. Although some useful information can be captured and conveyed with these qualifiers, the reader should appreciate the greater degree of subjectivity involved in these determinations than in the basic diagnosis.

Course specifiers, another group of specifiers, contrast a client's present status with his or her previous mental health history. In general, In Partial Remission means that full criteria were previously met, but only some of the original symptoms presently remain. In Full Remission means that there is currently a complete absence of symptoms, but that in the examiner's judgment it is clinically relevant to note the client's adjustment history. There is no absolute demarcation between In Full Remission and "Recovered" (when disorder would no longer be noted). Even when a client is judged to be Recovered, Prior History of a disorder can be noted if the examiner believes that this information has value for an understanding of the case. As an example, the literature on reading problems suggests that there may often be a history of developmental articulation problems that have been completely resolved in the backgrounds of poor readers. A diagnosis for such a child might be as follows:

Axis I   Reading Disorder
           Prior History of Phonological Disorder (recovered)
or
Axis I   Reading Disorder
           Phonological Disorder, In Full Remission

The distinction between these two is left up the examiner, but relevant variables may include the age of the child, the amount of time that has elapsed since criteria for Phonological Disorder were met, and where on the spectrum of "within normal limits" the child's current articulation falls.

For several disorders and their associated syndromes (Manic Episode, Major Depressive Episode, Substance Dependence), there are specific criteria for the qualifiers In Partial Remission and In Full Remission. For the Substance Dependence disorders, as an example, the course specifiers are Early Full Remission, Early Partial Remission, Sustained Full Remission, and Sustained Partial Remission. The qualifier Sustained Full Remission is used if there have been no symptoms of Substance Dependence or Substance Abuse for 12 months or longer. These course specifiers, however, are precluded by either of two additional specifiers: On Agonist Therapy or In a Controlled Environment. DSM-IV discusses the course specifiers for Substance Dependence on pages 179–180, and those for Mood Episodes on pages 387–391.

Also included on Axis I are behavior and situational problems that justify professional involvement but do not fall within the DSM-IV definition of mental disorder. As noted above, the class of Other Conditions That May Be a Focus Of Clinical Attention greatly expands the range of application of DSM-IV. Often called "V codes" (see the following Application Note), these conditions allow the examiner to address very real concerns in the lives of many children and adolescents—problems such as family conflict, physical or sexual abuse, unemployment, and identity issues. This section has been significantly expanded in DSM-IV, with a number of new categories available that were not present in DSM-III or DSM-III-R. The availability of categories for physical and sexual abuse and for neglect has been very helpful for child care specialists in many settings. Clinicians who address spiritual and religious concerns have, for the first time, an appropriate designation for these issues: V62.89, Religious or Spiritual Problems. In these and other instances, the availability of classification categories for research and clinical focus is very likely to promote further discussion and investigation (Turner, Lukoff, Barnhouse, & Lu, 1995). This is an extremely important section of DSM-IV for child and school psychologists to be familiar with.

APPLICATION NOTE   V Codes

The categories in the chapter "Other Conditions That May Be a Focus of Clinical Attention" are sometimes referred to as "V codes," because DSM-III and DSM-III-R all had ICD-9-CM numerical codes that began with the letter V. In DSM-IV, a number of categories have been added to this section that do not have ICD-9-CM numerical codes beginning with V; however, the general designation "V codes" continues to be used because it is more succinct than "Other Conditions . . . " and is clearly understood by almost all users.

Axis II: Personality Disorders and Mental Retardation

Although there seems to be some shared agreement as to what Axis II represents, the authors of DSM-IV have backed away from offering a formal defining statement. The text simply lists the types of information coded and/or noted on this axis: the Personality Disorders, Mental Retardation, notations of relevant personality traits (not coded), enduring defense mechanisms (not coded), and one of the V codes—Borderline Intellectual Functioning. Considering the diagnostic information included on Axis II, the reader will probably conclude that the intent is to reflect more enduring or stable aspects of the client's adjustment that affect his or her functioning. This indeed is the purpose of Axis II, but the precise differentiation of what should be considered Axis I and what Axis II has been problematic across DSM-III, DSM-III-R, and DSM-IV. DSM-III coded on Axis II only the Specific Developmental Disorders (roughly equivalent to DSM-IV Learning Disorders and some Communication Disorders) and the Personality Disorders (personality traits could also be noted but were not coded). DSM-III-R moved several DSM-III diagnoses from Axis I to Axis II, principally the Mental Retardation and Pervasive Developmental Disorders categories, which were grouped together with the Specific Developmental Disorders under the general heading of Developmental Disorders. (The Borderline Intellectual Functioning V code was also added to Axis II at this time.) All these disorders are often lifelong difficulties that arise early in childhood and can adversely affect multiple aspects of a client's life. The problems caused by this apparently reasonable modification was that it opened the Pandora's box of what the exact boundaries of Axes I and II were. The Attention Deficit Disorders (as they were then called), for instance, also arise early in childhood, and empirical evidence was accumulating that these too can be lifelong and pervasive patterns of disability. Other voices wondered whether early-onset Dysthymic Disorder—a longstanding pattern of low grade-depression—was not more similar to the Personality Disorders than to the Axis I Mood Disorders. With DSM-IV, the authors have retreated somewhat: Only Mental Retardation, Borderline Intellectual Functioning, and the Personality Disorder diagnoses are now coded on Axis II. Axis II can also be used to note associated personality traits or defense mechanisms, but there is no ICD-9-CM (numerical) coding of such observations and impressions. All other diagnoses are made on Axis I. When an Axis II diagnosis is the reason for the evaluation, this is noted by specifying "(Reason for Visit)" in an outpatient setting, or "(Primary Diagnosis)" in an inpatient setting, after the diagnosis.

The information on Axes I and II constitutes the mental health diagnosis proper. The remaining three axes are used to record additional information about the client that may provide a fuller understanding of his or her problems and situation. Only Axis I and II disorders have numerical codes linking these disorders with mental health conditions in the International Classification of Diseases, 9th revision, Clinical Modification (ICD-9-CM; World Health Organization, 1991) and Chapter V of the International Classification of Diseases, 10th revision (ICD-10; World Health Organization, 1992b). (Axis III disorders have numerical codes linking them with general medical conditions in ICD-9-CM.) Third-party carriers (insurance companies, Medicaid, the Social Security Administration) may or may not require information about the remaining three axes.

Axis III: General Medical Conditions

Provision for the inclusion of information about current physical disorders or conditions that are potentially relevant to the understanding or management of a case is the purpose of Axis III. These factors may or may not be etiological in nature (e.g., head injury associated with dementia [etiological] vs. diabetes as a clinical management issue in using food reinforcement with autistic child [nonetiological]). Axis III may be used to note associated physical findings of presumed importance (e.g., neurological "soft signs"). Sarma (1994) has a brief discussion of both minor physical anomalies and "minor neurological signs" (i.e., soft signs) of potential relevance to psychiatric disorders. For the purposes of DSM-IV, "General Medical Conditions" are the categories listed outside the "Mental and Behavioural Disorders" chapter (Chapter V) of ICD-9-CM/ICD-10.

For most nonmedically trained examiners, the use of Axis III is one of the most problematic aspects of applying DSM-IV. Yet the relevance of Axis III and its contribution to the understanding of an increasing number of childhood disorders can hardly be denied. Skodol (1989) discussed the use of Axis III by nonmedical mental health professionals and offered the opinion that notation on Axis III does not indicate that a particular diagnosis is being made by the person recording the multiaxial evaluation. He suggested that nonmedical clinicians may wish to indicate the sources of their information on Axis III. This simple convention will reduce the anxiety of most examiners about using Axis III and prevent any professional concerns about nonphysicians' diagnosing a medical illness (see the following Professional Note).

PROFESSIONAL NOTE   The Use of Axis III
by the Nonphysician

I would recommend as best practice that the school psychologist or
other nonmedical professional indicated the sources of all Axis III
information or determinations, as in these examples:

Axis III   Mother reported that child has juvenile onset diabetes.
Axis III   Genetic karyotype indicates trisomy 21.
Axis III   Seizure disorder diagnosed by child's pediatrician, James
Lee, M.D.

Axis IV: Psychosocial and Environmental Problems

Axis IV is used to list psychological, social, and environmental problems that contribute to a client's problems and adjustment. The DSM-
III and DSM-III-R versions of Axis IV called for a rating on a multipoint
scale. The current version simply has the examiner list environmental information that is judged clinically relevant to the development
or exacerbation of a mental disorder, or that has itself become the
focus of clinical intervention. Nine general categories for consideration are offered, and the examiner is asked to specify the exact circumstances causing stress for the child (see p. 30 of DSM-IV). The
index period for consideration is typically the past year, but the examiner is given ample discretion to consider more distant events if
this contributes to an understanding of the case. For certain specific
disorders (e.g., Posttraumatic Stress Disorder), it may be necessary to
include information on events prior to the past year.

Axis V: Global Assessment of Functioning

The Global Assessment of Functioning (GAF) rating on Axis V reflects the examiner's overall judgment of the child's mental health
and adjustment on a 0–100 ordinal scale (see p. 32 of DSM-IV). GAF
ratings are based on psychological, social, and school (or occupational) functioning; environmental circumstances, opportunities, and
deprivations are not considered in making GAF ratings. GAF ratings
are usually made for the current time, but can also be made for the
highest period of functioning over the past year (this may be prog-

nostic of a child's or adolescent's eventual outcome) or any other specified period or point. Global assessment scales were included in the two previous editions of DSM and derive from a empirical and clinical literature that supports their reliability, validity, and utility (Goldman, Skodol, & Lave, 1992). Axis V provides an opportunity for the evaluator to give a summary assessment of the client's level of adjustment. This can be very valuable for tracking the progress of a child or adolescent, assessing response to treatment, and documenting subtle changes in status. The scale provides for placement on a range from superior adjustment to totally compromised failure to adapt. In this particular aspect of using DSM-IV, a novice may find discussion and review of cases with colleagues an especially useful training experience. In my course on using the DSM, the classroom discussions concerning appropriate GAF ratings clearly provide a kind of norming of this scale.

A convention I have found useful is to identify the global category that appears to summarize a child's or adolescent's adjustment best. If the young person clearly falls within this category, I might give him or her a central rating (e.g., 65); if he or she seems to be approaching the next category up or down, a rating near the boundary is given (e.g., 69 or 61). I routinely indicate positive (and negative) changes in increments of 2 (e.g., from 65 to 67), because this gives room to report a mild regression at the next evaluation that still leaves the child doing better than the original review (66). The use of Axis V is one of the aspects of DSM-IV where the critical role of an examiner's clinical judgment becomes clear; there is no absolute criterion or "gold standard" by which the accuracy of GAF ratings can be evaluated. These ratings represent the examiner's best professional judgment at the time.

The current GAF measure is scaled through the combination of several different elements that have qualitatively different weights: the number and severity of symptoms, the environmental consequences of these symptoms, and the risk they pose for loss of life or self-determination. Certain critical events (e.g., a suicide attempt) drive the rating very low, even in the context of otherwise adequate signs of functioning. The presence of "symptoms" is first noted regarding GAF ratings of 70 or below. In almost all cases, the diagnosis of any mental disorder is associated with an Axis V rating at or below 70, because of this feature. However, the converse is not always true: The remission of a mental disorder does not automatically mean that a client's GAF rating will be above 70. It is the impression of some evaluators that certain third-party carriers use Axis V as part of their determination regarding qualification for reimbursement (i.e., that only claims with

GAF ratings at or below 70 are judged to be covered by mental health provisions). I bring up this belief only to make a critical point that will be discussed more fully later: GAF ratings—indeed, the entire DSM-IV diagnosis—must be made only with respect to the case data available. Axis V is based on a child's or adolescent's psychological, social, and academic functioning, not on whether the young person's family will be covered by any medical insurance the family may have.

PRECEDENCE OF DIAGNOSES: DIAGNOSTIC CONVENTIONS, HIERARCHIES, AND MULTIPLE DIAGNOSES

In general, DSM-IV actively encourages multiple diagnoses, so that the salient problems experienced by a client can be fully described. This is one of the clearest contrasts between the approach taken to classification by the DSM committee and that taken by the authors of the ICD classification. The philosophy of ICD-9 (World Health Organization, 1977) appeared to encourage as much parsimony as possible in diagnosis. This may change with ICD-10, which appears to accept the possibility of a client's needing multiple diagnoses more readily (World Health Organization, 1992a, 1992b). The DSM philosophy from DSM-III onward has been to encourage multiple diagnoses, so that the full complexities of each individual case can be captured to the extent possible.

Some diagnostic possibilities, however, take precedence over others. Three general considerations bearing upon multiple diagnoses are used to bring order to the potential chaos of uncontrolled proliferation of diagnoses in a given case. Each of these three exceptions is associated with several standard phrases found repeatedly in the text of DSM-IV, and coming to recognize these "directions" will go a long way toward decreasing the confusion many new users feel in trying to make sense of the language of the DSM-IV text. The three general circumstances of diagnostic precedence that exercise some restrictions on the usual practice of making multiple diagnoses are these: (1) The symptoms are associated features of a more pervasive disorder; (2) the symptoms are due to a general medical condition or to substance use; and (3) the symptoms represent a "boundary zone" of uncertainty between two diagnostic formulations.

In the most commonly encountered possibility, certain symptoms that potentially could be diagnosed as a recognized syndrome are seen as associated features of a more pervasive disorder. More pervasive, generalized patterns of disturbance usually take diagnostic precedence over more specific, focal difficulties if the narrow-band problems develop within the context of the more generalized difficulty. For example, the disorder Schizophrenia often includes symptoms of chronic depression, anhedonia, and poor self-esteem; all of these are also symptoms of Dysthymic Disorder. These mood symptoms are not used to identify the syndrome of Schizophrenia and are not part of the diagnostic criteria of Schizophrenia, but are discussed as "associated symptoms." The position of DSM-IV is that a separate diagnosis of Dysthymic Disorder should not be made in an individual who has received a diagnosis of Schizophrenia, because these symptoms are so commonly linked with the problem (even if they are not used as diagnostic criteria). The phrases used in the text to alert the user to this consideration are "has never met the criteria for . . . ," "does not meet the criteria for . . . ," and "does not occur exclusively during the course of . . . ."

There are, however, exceptions to the general rule of subsuming associated problems under the diagnosis of a more generalized problem. For example, sleep problems are common in Depressive Disorders, and insomnia is a criterion symptom of the Major Depression syndrome in DSM-IV, which forms the basis for the Major Depressive Disorder diagnosis. Insomnia associated with Major Depressive Disorder is usually considered only a symptom of the depression. Nevertheless, an independent diagnosis of a Sleep Disorder is allowed in conjunction with Major Depressive Disorder under certain conditions. If the sleep problem is the predominant complaint being evaluated and is clinically significant enough to warrant independent treatment, a separate classification is made. The diagnosis would be Insomnia Related to Major Depressive Disorder (Primary Diagnosis) and Major Depressive Disorder.

A second general rule of diagnostic formulation throughout DSM-IV is that when any problem is considered to be a manifestation of a known biological illness or chemical influence, these influences take precedence in diagnosis. The key phrase seen often in DSM-IV is "not due to the direct physiological effects of a substance (e.g., a drug of abuse, or a medication) or a general medical condition." This tells the reader that these conditions preempt the diagnosis of other mental disorders. Symptoms of depression that arise as a consequence of Alcohol Abuse, for instance, should not be diagnosed as Major Depressive Disorder but as Alcohol-Induced Mood Disorder.

The third general directive pertains to circumstances where a given clinical situation could possibly be accounted for by two different diagnoses. In such circumstances the examiner must review all the data available and make a determination as to which diagnosis best represents a client's situation. The text phrase used to alert the reader to possible alternative conceptualizations is this: "is not better accounted for by . . . ."

CHILD AND ADOLESCENT
MENTAL HEALTH AND DSM-IV

Our understanding of mental health problems in children and adolescents lags behind the level of knowledge that has been achieved with adults. Several factors have contributed to this disparity, and some of these continue to operate. For many decades, emotional and behavioral problems in young people were treated solely as juvenile extensions of the difficulties seen in adults, with little or no appreciation of the unique developmental features of childhood and adolescence that can affect the forms psychopathology takes. The research methods necessitated by these developmental features (e.g., large-scale, longitudinal studies and naturalistic observation methodologies) are often time-consuming, labor-intensive, and expensive— factors that have further slowed progress. For research involving some degree of risk (intervention studies or intensive assessment investigations), there is an understandable caution about conducting research on young people, but this also has the cost of slowing our learning. Finally, there is a real possibility that psychopathology in the rapidly changing child or adolescent is to some degree a different phenomenon from that seen in the more consistently behaving adult. The behavior of children and adolescents changes as they learn, grow, and develop. Clearly, some patterns of psychopathology change over time, but possibly the very construct of mental disorder in young people refers to more fluid and less consistent manifestations than those seen in adults, who generally have established life routines.

Considering all these factors, it is not too surprising that the formulations of behavioral and emotional problems affecting children and adolescents have tended to show great change with each subsequent edition of the DSM. It is no great leap of inference to anticipate that this will continue into DSM-V. The reasoned application of DSM-IV to the complexities of child and adolescent adjustment is a challenging intellectual and clinical activity.

For the practicing school psychologist or other child psychologist, one of the most important aspects in learning to use DSM-IV accurately is to recognize that there is no "child section" of DSM-IV nor are there "child diagnoses." The clear position of the American Psychiatric Association from DSM-III thorough DSM-III-R to DSM-IV has been that basic mental health phenomena are essentially the same, regardless of age or developmental stage. For example, the manifestation and experience of severe depression are seen as very similar in children, in adolescents, in adults, and in geriatric populations. There is some recognition of age-associated features, but these are seen as minor variations on the major themes. Similarly, there is no separate discussion of "Childhood Schizophrenia" as a separate taxonomic category from Schizophrenia in adults. The core symptoms of the disorder labeled Schizophrenia are seen as basically the same, regardless of an individual's age; developmental features provide some secondary elaborations of these manifestations, but do not change the essential equation. One consequence of this formulation is that the school psychologist must be just as familiar with the entire text of DSM-IV as the psychologist who usually sees adult or geriatric populations. There is no child section or chapter from which the school psychologist can safely assume that all his or her diagnostic decisions will originate.

There is a problem, however, because the structure of DSM-IV creates the *illusion* for the occasional user that there is a child section. As was the case in DSM-III and DSM-III-R, the first chapter of diagnostic categories in DSM-IV specifically refers to youth: "Disorders Usually First Diagnosed in Infancy, Childhood, or Adolescence" (DSM-IV); "Disorders Usually First Evident in Infancy, Childhood, or Adolescence" (DSM-III and DSM-III-R). It is the only nonthematic grouping of diagnoses. That is, these diagnoses are placed together not because they share basic similarities in character (e.g., they all involve problems with mood regulation or are associated with substance use), but because they tend to be first diagnosed prior to adulthood. These diagnoses are *not* restricted to use with children and adolescents (a common misperception). Adults may be assigned these diagnoses; indeed, many of these diagnoses could be given for the first time in adulthood (this is not common, but it is possible). By constituting this chapter on a very different basis from that of all other chapters, the authors of DSM-III and subsequent editions created a number of difficulties.

One problem was that some diagnoses from this early-onset group seemed virtually identical to disorders in the Anxiety Disorders group (e.g., Overanxious Disorder [DSM-III and DSM-III-R] vs. Generalized Anxiety Disorder [DSM-III, DSM-III-R, and DSM-IV]). This has been resolved in DSM-IV by subsuming Overanxious Disorder under Generalized Anxiety Disorder. A second type of problem was the splitting up of thematic groups by pulling some diagnoses into the first chapter because of the ages when they were often first diagnosed. For example, there was an Anxiety Disorders group in DSM-III-R, and there was an Anxiety Disorders of Childhood grouping in the first chapter; there was a Sexual Disorders group in DSM-III-R, and there was a Gender Identity Disorders group in the first chapter. This second problem has been reduced but not totally eliminated in DSM-IV. One anxiety problem has been left in the first chapter (Separation Anxiety Disorder); an "Eating Disorders" chapter has been set up, but three specific eating problems have been left in the first chapter (Pica, Rumination Disorder, and Feeding Disorder of Infancy or Early Childhood). This dual representation of diagnostic topics is a continuing source of confusion for the users of DSM-IV. A final problem is the impression of some users that children should be diagnosed with disorders from the first chapter and that consideration of the rest of the text has limited relevance in conceptualizing maladjustment of childhood. This view is mistaken. The only answer to this continuing difficulty is continuing education regarding the broad outline of DSM-IV, so that all potentially relevant diagnostic categories can be considered.

◆

See DSM-IV-TR Coding Note: The GAF Rating in DSM-IV-TR, in 2002 Updates, page 234.

CHAPTER 3

♦♦♦

Learning to Use DSM-IV

♦

CATEGORICAL CLASSIFICATION

The most important information for each diagnosis in DSM-IV is found in the sentence that begins: "The essential feature(s) of [Name of Disorder or Class of Disorders] is . . . ." This statement provides the conceptual foundation for the diagnosis. The diagnostic criteria for each specific diagnosis (or group of diagnoses) document different patterns of manifestation *within the context identified by the essential feature.* The essential feature, then is like a street address of a particular friend, but first the examiner needs to be sure that he or she is in the right "city." This is illustrated by the final diagnosis given in most sections and chapters: the Not Otherwise Specified (NOS) option. An important and positive change in DSM-IV has been the addition of NOS options to several groups of diagnoses often used with children and adolescents. The NOS option lists no diagnostic criteria and is sometimes disparagingly described as a "blank check" that evaluators can use to give any diagnosis that they please without being bothered by the restrictions of diagnostic criteria. This is not a valid view of the application of an NOS diagnosis. Such a diagnosis is properly applied when an evaluator has concluded that the particular case is best understood as an instance of the general problem area identified—that is, that a child's or adolescent's problems are best captured within a group of difficulties sharing an essential feature.

Let me illustrate this difference in orientation. Within the "Disorders Usually First Diagnosed in Infancy, Childhood, or Adolescence" chapter is the section on Attention-Deficit and Disruptive Behavior Disorders; these disorders include the category Attention-Deficit/

Hyperactivity Disorder (ADHD) and the category Attention-Deficit/ Hyperactivity Disorder Not Otherwise Specified (ADHD NOS). This section begins as follows: "The essential feature of Attention-Deficit/ Hyperactivity Disorder is a persistent pattern of inattention and/or hyperactivity–impulsivity that is more frequent and severe than is typically observed in individuals at a comparable level of development (Criterion A)" (p. 78). The basic ADHD category contains three subtypes based on various combinations of symptoms from the ADHD criteria set. The ADHD NOS category involves a single line of text: "This category is for disorders with prominent symptoms of inattention or hyperactivity–impulsivity that do not meet criteria for Attention-Deficit/Hyperactivity Disorder" (p. 85). The examiner is free to use the ADHD NOS category to diagnose children (or adults) who do not meet the various criteria for ADHD. The expectation in doing this is that the problematic pattern of behavior and adjustment being considered *does* include the essential feature of the category being considered and that this is the best organizing principle for the available data. The NOS option gives the evaluator a significant degree of freedom, but it also places a significant burden on him or her to use the system in a responsible and appropriate manner. The authors of DSM-IV make the point that the classification system is not intended to be applied in a rigid, "cookbook" manner that reduces the professional to a technician (p. xxiii). This point is directly relevant to the use of the NOS diagnoses.

DIFFERENTIAL DIAGNOSIS

The primary task of the school psychologist or other professional examiner using DSM-IV to diagnose a child or adolescent is to determine which category or categories best capture the nature of the young person's current problems in adjustment and functioning. The presenting concerns that bring the youth to the examiner's attention could potentially be signs of several different patterns of maladjustment. For instance, a teacher's report that a child exhibits aggressive behavior during recess and class changes might indicate an Adjustment Disorder, a Mood Disorder, Conduct Disorder, or some other diagnosis. The collection of additional data regarding the child, the child's history of problems, and his or her concomitant difficulties allows a rational choice to be made among the various diagnostic possibilities. "Ruling in" (identifying) or "ruling out" (excluding from consideration; see the following Application Note) different categories is known as the process of "differential diagnosis." The text iden-

APPLICATION NOTE "Rule Out"

The phrase "rule out" does not appear in DSM-IV and is not part of the vocabulary of DSM. However, it is a common expression in psychiatric diagnosis and is often seen in reports, especially from professionals with medical training or experience in medical settings. There is often some confusion among nonphysicians as to the meaning of this expression. "Rule out" is typically used to identify an alternative diagnosis that is being actively considered, but for which sufficient data has not yet been obtained. For instance, the diagnostic statement "Alcohol Abuse, rule out Alcohol Dependence," suggests that the examiner has definitely concluded there is a drinking problem; that there is definitely evidence supporting Alcohol Abuse; and that the more serious problem of Alcohol Dependence may be present, but the available evidence is inconclusive. "Rule out" can be thought of as a reminder or instruction to continue seeking the information which would allow a diagnosis to be conclusively identified or eliminated from consideration (for the present).

---

tifies for most major diagnoses which alternative conceptualizations are most likely to be considered, and it attempts to highlight relevant differences.

The new user of DSM-IV may be somewhat overwhelmed by these sections of the manual; to many of us, it initially appears that "everything is a differential diagnosis for everything." With only a little experience, however, certain underlying relationships become more familiar and the process of differential diagnosis becomes more selective. Appendix A of DSM-IV (pp. 689–701) offers decision trees for six major areas: Mental Disorders Due to a General Medical Condition, Substance-Induced Disorders, Psychotic Disorders, Mood Disorders, Anxiety Disorders, and Somatoform Disorders. I have found that these decision trees, in addition to guiding consideration of particular cases, are useful in helping novices to gain an overall appreciation for the structure of DSM-IV.

ORDERING OF DIAGNOSES

When multiple diagnoses are made, the accepted convention is that the diagnoses are listed in order of clinical importance or anticipated clinical attention. The first diagnosis listed usually also pertains to the reason for the evaluation. This is the conceptualization or understanding of the presenting problem(s) that led to the assessment. In some cases, however, the first (most significant) diagnosis will not be the reason for the evaluation. In these instances, the manual directs noting "(Principal Diagnosis)" or "(Reason for Visit)" after the diagnosis associated with the referral (see the following Application Note). When the reason for the evaluation is an Axis I diagnosis, it is assumed that this is the first diagnosis unless noted otherwise. If the reason for the evaluation is an Axis II condition, this is noted as in this example:

Axis I   Tourette's Disorder
Axis II   Mental Retardation, Mild (Reason for Visit)

DEGREE OF DIAGNOSTIC CONFIDENCE

The manual allows for varying degrees of confidence versus uncertainty in the diagnosis arrived at. In an uncertain case, a diagnosis can be given, followed by the specifier "(Provisional)." For example, a diagnosis of Oppositional Defiant Disorder requires a pattern of at least four of eight symptoms of hostile, negativistic, noncompliant behavior over at least 6 months. If I saw clear evidence of three of the eight symptoms, and thought there was an indication of a fourth symp-

---

APPLICATION NOTE   "(Principal Diagnosis)"/"(Reason for Visit)"

In identifying which of several diagnoses given is the reason for the evaluation, there are two conventions. First, if nothing further is specified, then it is assumed that the Axis I diagnosis listed first corresponds to the reason for assessment. If another Axis I diagnosis or an Axis II diagnosis is the reason for the contact, this is noted with one of two phrases: "(Reason for Visit)" in an outpatient setting or "(Principal Diagnosis)" in a hospital or other inpatient setting. "(Principal Diagnosis)" identifies the reason for a hospital admission when a child or adolescent has several diagnoses and the decision to hospitalize the young person is not based on the diagnosis listed first on Axis I. Despite this differentation in the text, the reader will quickly discover that the phrase "(Principal Diagnosis)" is often used by many professionals in both inpatient and outpatient settings to mark the reason for the contact.

---

tom but did not have clear documentation of it, I might give "Oppositional Defiant Disorder (Provisional)" as my diagnosis. The key point in using "(Provisional)" is this: The examiner believes that the required characteristics *are* probably present and that further data will substantiate this. This can be contrasted with the use of Disruptive Behavior Disorder NOS. In this latter diagnosis the examiner is convinced that there is evidence of a mental disorder, and that the general type of mental disorder meets the essential features of a Disruptive Behavior Disorder; however, the examiner is not convinced that additional information will conform to the pattern of Oppositional Defiant Disorder. The discussion on pages 3–5 of DSM-IV covers the major ways to indicate degree of diagnostic uncertainty.

HOW TO RECORD DIAGNOSES

Diagnostic categories in DSM-IV are defined by diagnostic criteria and identified by titles (e.g., Bulimia Nervosa). Associated with each diagnostic category is also a four- or five- digit number—three digits followed by either one or two decimal places (e.g., 307.51). The numeral is the *International Classification of Diseases*, 9th revision, Clinical Modification (ICD-9-CM) code for the particular Mental Disorder. This is found with the title for a diagnostic category (e.g., "307.51 Bulimia Nervosa," p. 545) and with the diagnostic criteria (e.g., "Diagnostic criteria for 307.51 Bulimia Nervosa," p. 549). In addition, the titles and ICD-9-CM codes for all diagnoses are given in the summary overview ("DSM-IV Classification," pp. 13–24), Appendix E ("Alphabetical List of DSM-IV Diagnoses and Codes," pp. 793–802), and Appendix F ("Numerical Listing of DSM-IV Diagnoses and Codes," pp. 803–812).

All DSM-IV diagnoses are legitimate ICD-9-CM diagnoses, but this does not mean that all DSM-IV categories can be found in ICD-9-CM. A review of Appendix F reveals that a number of DSM-IV diagnoses have the same numerical code; that is, some of the differentiations made in DSM-IV are collapsed into a single ICD-9-CM category. Similarity, there are diagnoses available in ICD-9-CM that do not appear in DSM-IV. The DSM-IV NOS diagnoses for the relevant problem areas are often used to diagnose these cases. As another example, a greater selection of "V codes" (diagnostic categories that are not Mental Disorders but may be of clinical importance) is available in ICD-9-CM than in DSM-IV. All submissions for insurance or government reimbursement must be made in terms of the ICD-9-CM numerical codes, but these are included in DSM-IV, and for most purposes it is not necessary for a school psychologist to have a copy of ICD-9-CM.

Sometime, probably in the first decade of the 21st century, the U.S. Department of Health and Human Services will begin requiring the use of codes from the *International Classification of Diseases,* 10th revision (ICD-10). Several versions of ICD-10 have already been published. It will significantly expand the number of available codes, both for Mental Disorders and for General Medical Conditions. The mechanics of this expansion of categories will involve a shift from pure numerical codes (001–999) to alphanumerical codes (A00 to Z99). Most of the codes pertaining to mental health problems will still be found in Chapter V, but these codes will begin with the letter F (rather than falling between 290 and 319, as they do in ICD-9). Bulimia Nervosa, for instance, will be coded as F50.2 in ICD-10. All DSM-IV categories will be legitimate diagnoses in ICD-10, although, again, there will not be perfect correspondence. ICD-10, for example, will have a diagnostic category "Bulimia nervosa, atypical, F50.3" (World Health Organization, 1992b) that is not found in DSM-IV. (It would probably be classified as Eating Disorder NOS.) Appendix H of DSM-IV, "DSM-IV Classification With ICD-10 Codes" (pp. 829–841), gives the codes that will be used for reporting and reimbursement submission when the shift to ICD-10 is made in the United States. A revised printing of DSM-IV will no doubt be issued at that point for those who do not wish to keep turning to the back of the text for the proper code.

INTERPRETATION OF DIAGNOSTIC IMPRESSIONS FROM OTHER SOURCES

Because the goal of a diagnostic classification is to communicate as much information about a child or adolescent as possible, it is valuable in making such a classification to take into consideration the information conveyed by other professionals in their diagnostic formulations. The school psychologist is often in the position of analyzing data from a variety of sources and perspectives. These data routinely include the reports of parents, teachers, and other adults working in a school setting, as well as scores on behavior rating scales, results of academic achievement testing in the classroom, grades, and interviews with the child. However, they also increasingly include reports from child care professionals outside the school system. Independent psychological evaluations from clinical or school psychologists; speech and audiology reports; discharge summaries or case notes from neurologists, neurosurgeons, and psychiatrists; social history reports from juvenile court officers; chemical dependence program evaluations—all of these may become part of the school psychologist's data base for a child or adolescent. Some of these professionals will use the format of DSM-IV to communicate their summary impressions of the child's situation; others will pass along impressions from third-party sources expressed in the language of DSM. Many school psychologists will already be familiar with the wide variability of practice in the clinical use of DSM-IV among child care professionals from a variety of disciplines. This can be a motivating influence for each of us to be as clear as possible in our own diagnostic formulations and to document the data we believe indicate the signs and symptoms supporting these diagnostic impressions.

Occasionally, when in reviewing old records, an examiner will need to deal with diagnoses from DSM-III or DSM-III-R. Appendix D in DSM-IV, "Annotated Listing of Changes in DSM-IV" (pp. 773–791), gives a general discussion of the alterations in diagnostic categories between these two versions. Appendix D of DSM-III-R, "Annotated Comparative Listing of DSM-III and DSM-III-R" (pp. 409–430 there), served the same purpose. I continue to find it valuable on occasion to have copies of both DSM-III and DSM-III-R available in my office.

PART II

◆◆◆

GUIDELINES FOR EVALUATION OF PRESENTING PROBLEMS

◆

Evaluation of a child or adolescent referred for psychological services begins with the presenting problems that have brought the young person to professional attention. Most often, the youth's adult caretakers have voiced some concerns regarding his or her actions, performance, and/or emotions. Thus begins the process of diagnostic formulation. Presenting concerns both raise diagnostic possibilities and suggest areas of investigation to refine diagnostic hypotheses. As further data are gathered, the clinical picture of the young person's adjustment is developed in greater and greater detail. The goal of diagnostic classification is to recognize the most important patterns within the assessment data and to assign these the diagnosis or diagnoses that capture the most helpful information about the child's or adolescent's adjustment, functioning, and problems.

In this part of the book, some of the most common presenting concerns of caretakers are reviewed with respect to how DSM-IV diagnoses can be assigned to these. The organization of this discussion is thematic. Beginning with a broad area of concern—that is, acting-out or externalizing behavior problems—the diagnostic categories of potential relevance are discussed. Initial consideration is usually given to the most salient categories or the ones most frequently applied; alternative possibilities with lower base rates are then discussed in turn. Usually, possible diagnoses drawn from multiple chapters within DSM-IV are reviewed, because a human problem is seldom so simple and straightforward that one and only one diagnostic formation will be apparent from the first contact. A common source of confusion and frustration among my first-year graduate students as they begin to learn the DSM-IV system is that "You have to know it all just to begin." The examiner does need a general familiarity with the total classification system and with the logic of the system, because differential diagnoses from several areas within DSM-IV may need to be considered for each case. DSM-IV itself tries to address this difficulty with the "Differential Diagnosis" section for each diagnosis. The text by First, Frances, and Pincus (1995) draws together material on differential diagnostic considerations and organizes this in several ways, in order to assist the evaluator in considereing the most likely choices and to highlight the critical points of difference among these. I hope that the organization of the present book helps the reader develop a rapid familiarity with the DSM-IV framework, and that this understanding will assist in the efficient use of the classification system.

To help accomplish this goal, it has been necessary to keep the text relatively brief. This has been accomplished in several ways. Some of the discussions of specific diagnoses are quite brief, even when a great deal is known about the pattern, course, and variant expressions of a problem. In fact, especially when a great deal is known about a problem and it is generally well understood by most practicing psychologists, this common knowledge is not reiterated. The purpose here is not to give a general discussion of behavioral and emotional problems in youth. There are several good texts on child psychopathology; in particular, Kronenberger and Meyer (1996) use DSM-IV as the framework for discussing the assessment and treatment of childhood problems. In this part of the present book, I describe the categories of DSM-IV, attempt to clarify the diagnostic issues onvolved, and show how clinical information can be represented within DSM-IV.

Another departure from many professional presentations is that referencing is intentionally sparse. Relatively noncontroversial statements regarding behavior problems are simply presented. The references that are given have usually been selected because they provide particularly pertinent results, because they represent recent empirical research, or occasionally because of their classic status within the history of psychology. Opinions and conclusions based on my personal professional experience are identified as such to the best of my ability.

CHAPTER 4

◆◆◆

Disruptive Behavior Symptoms (Externalizing Problems)

◆

OVERVIEW

Familiar to school psychologists is the finding that the most frequent basis for a mental health referral from teachers or parents is some pattern of rule-defiant behaviors (Shamsie & Hluchy, 1991). Doll's (1996) review of epidemiological studies found DSM-III and DSM-III-R behavioral disorders (Conduct Disorder [CD], Oppositional Disorder or Oppositional Defiant Disorder [ODD], and Attention Deficit Disorder [ADD] or Attention-deficit Hyperactivity Disorder [ADHD]) to be among the most frequently diagnosed psychiatric disorders in school children. Various labels have been used in the psychological literature to describe children who disobey adults, act in violation of understood expectations within a setting, attack their peers, and disrupt the cooperation of others in play or work. At the turn of the century, the term "conduct problems" began to be used with increasing frequency. Psychodynamic writers spoke of "acting-out behavior." Empirical analyses of the covariations between "externalizing" behaviors appeared. Advocates of behavior modification tended to speak of "oppositional behavior." Increasing empirical evidence began to accumulate that such problems are persistent, often get worse instead of better over time, and predict multiple negative outcomes for a child. Further reports brought increasing awareness that these problems are often difficult to treat, and that traditional interventions have very limited usefulness. Eventually empirical confirmation became available for what clinicians had feared: These behavior problems are associated with other serious problems— substance misuse and adult personality disturbances. Disruptive behavior problems remain among the most challenging areas of service for psychologists and other child care professionals.

Disruptive behavior problems in school settings manifest themselves in repeated conflictual encounters with peers, teachers, and other school personnel. Children with these problems are the ones most frequently corrected or reprimanded for their public behavior. They are usually well known to the school secretary, the custodian, and the playground supervisor. Disruptive behavior problems can be situational but more typically occur across all of a child's environments, especially those which call for self-control, cooperative behavior, turn taking, and restraint in movement and activity. These problems tend to be overt and obvious to the adults in each setting (although the behaviors may not be perceived as "mental health problems"). Moreover, there can be relatively good correspondence between the reports of children with disruptive behavior problems and the reports of adults regarding them (Cantwell, Lewinsohn, Rohde, & Seeley, 1997). However, whether such children qualify for services under the Individuals with Disabilities Education Act (IDEA) is far less obvious and is a matter of continuing debate (see the next two IDEA Notes).

Several groups of DSM-IV diagnoses deal with oppositional, rule-defiant, and aggressive behavior. First et al. (1995) give differential diagnosis decision trees for aggressive behavior, behavior problems in a child or adolescent, and the Mental Disorder categories most commonly seen in disruptive and impulse control syndromes. Among the differential diagnoses to be considered with these presenting concerns are the following (see below for further discussion):

Conduct Disorder
Oppositional Defiant Disorder
Attention-Deficit/Hyperactivity Disorder
Bipolar I Disorder, Most Recent Manic Episode
Intermittent Explosive Disorder
Adjustment Disorder With Disturbance of Conduct
Personality Change Due to [neurological injury or illness]; Disinhibited Type, Aggressive Type, or Combined Type

In addition to establishing the clearest diagnostic classification of a child's or adolescent's presenting concerns, the examiner should carefully consider any associated behavior problems the youth may be experiencing. Disruptive behavior problems tend to have high comorbidities with other psychiatric problems. As always, the general issue is how to "capture" all relevant clinical information about a young

IDEA NOTE   Disruptive Behavior Disorders and IDEA

The diagnostic categories of DSM-IV do not automatically correspond to the eligibility categories identified in IDEA. Even when identical labels are used, the precise definitions (or absence of definitions) often leave open serious questions regarding the equivalence of the behavior problems outlined in the two systems. The Disruptive Behavior Disorders (CD, ODD, and Disruptive Behavior Disorder Not Otherwise Specified [NOS]) would seem to fall within the area identified in IDEA as "seriously emotionally disturbed" (behavior disorder). (For a separate discussion of ADHD and IDEA, see the IDEA note on p. 54.) One major emphasis in IDEA is a focus on disability conditions that handicap a child in achieving academic or vocational success. The increased attention in DSM-IV to the functional impairment criteria in almost all diagnoses criteria has obvious relevance here. The Global Assessment of Functioning (GAF) rating on Axis V also bears on this aspect of comparison. Mental disorders with symptoms that directly interfere with academic achievement or social development will be easier to establish as relevant for IDEA classification. Very low GAF scores associated with severe manifestations of mental disorders will also help document the handicaps needed for IDEA.

The essential feature of CD consists of repeated major rule violations and acts against the basic rights of others. The symptoms and consequences of CD will almost always easily support a classification under the "serious emotional disturbance" description category of IDEA. In my opinion, a strong case can usually be made for ODD and for Disruptive Behavior Disorder NOS, given the serious and chronic nature of these problems; however, more efforts to document the effects of these disorders upon scholastic achievement will be necessary to carry this case forward.

What is most important for the reader to recognize is that the categories of IDEA and DSM-IV do not automatically translate into each other. The basic purpose, structure, and methods of the two systems are different, and the "mapping" of one upon the other is imperfect and open to differences of interpretation. I believe that establishing an objective case for a mental disorder diagnosis will usually support and facilitate qualification of a student as eligible for services under IDEA. Furthermore, the establishment of several classifications in DSM-IV that are not mental disorders (the V codes) can also serve as a basis for seeking special services under IDEA. Psychiatric classification can help document intellectual, personal, and social problems that limit a young person's success in school and in the community; this opens the door for eligibility under IDEA. (However, see the IDEA Note on p. 44 for cautions about IDEA eligibility in such cases.)

IDEA NOTE   Cautions about Disruptive Behavior Disorders and IDEA

Considerable confusion and disagreement have surrounded the inclusion of children with serious conduct problems under IDEA. The definition of "seriously emotionally disturbed" in IDEA contains an exclusion for children whose behavior is "socially maladjusted" but does not fall within the conditions defined as "seriously emotionally disturbed." Unfortunately, no definition of "socially maladjusted" is given, so it is not clear what has been excluded. The usual interpretation is that delinquent behavior in isolation does not qualify a child as eligible for special services unless that child also meets one or more of the conditions identified as "seriously emotionally disturbed." Of some importance is that the act clearly does not exclude children who are "socially maladjusted"; it only indicates that social maladjustment alone is insufficient to establish eligibility under IDEA. Even more unfortunately, some state policies have been written to use DSM diagnoses of CD or ODD for exclusion from qualification under IDEA. Such a position would appear to be counter to the intention of the act (Cline, 1990; Council for Children with Behavioral Disorders, 1987) and at odds with the populations often served by special education (McGinnis, 1986).

---

person and his or her problems and situation most effectively and efficiently. Among the frequently reported comorbid conditions for many of the disruptive problems are the following:

Mood Disorders
Anxiety Disorders
Learning Disorders
Elimination Disorders (Enuresis, Encopresis)
Communication Disorders
Substance Use Disorders (usually in adolescence)

In addition to formal diagnoses, other pertinent individual differences can be recorded within the framework of DSM-IV. Two such characteristics of relevance to disruptive behavior problems are early temperament and intelligence. The potential importance of early temperamental differences among children in the development of behavior problems is increasingly being recognized. As I have noted in Chapter 2, Axis II can be used to record noncategorical information regarding personality traits and other characterological information. A child's intelligence is another variable that appears to interact with a history of behavior problems to affect prognosis; in general, higher intelligence appears to be associated with a better prognosis for later successful adjustment in children with such problems. Data about intellectual ability can also be noted on Axis II, even if it does not involve a diagnostic classification.

A childhood history of disruptive behavior problems has been associated with a number of serious adult diagnoses—notably Antisocial Personality Disorder, Borderline Personality Disorder, and Schizophrenia. Moreover, disruptive children are at high risk of social adjustment problems in adulthood even when they do not qualify for mental health diagnoses; marital conflict, child abuse, occupational maladjustment, and legal problems are overrepresented in their follow-up evaluations. In general, it is not safe to assume that these children will grow out of their problems in adjusting to the expectations of others and of society.

Finally, a number of pathological environmental circumstances are overrepresented in the lives of many youth with disruptive behavior problems. The examiner should be alert to the presence in a child's or adolescent's environment of abuse, neglect, and/or modeling of antisocial attitudes and behavior. A family history of criminal behavior, substance abuse, or mood disorders may contribute to the environmental adversity often seen in the backgrounds of the children. One concern expressed by Power and DuPaul (1996b) in their review of the ADHD categories of DSM-IV is that because the medical model conceptualizes the problem behavior as a manifestation of a disorder within a child, this may reduce an examiner's sensitivity to environmental factors that influence the conflicts between the child and his or her caretaking situations. It is absolutely the case that DSM-IV does explicitly conceptualize ADHD and all other mental disorders as disorders of the individual. It is not inevitable that taking such a view will lead one to ignore or minimize the powerful role played by setting variables and contingencies of consequences, but examiners are well cautioned to be sure to take these influences into consideration.

DIFFERENTIAL DIAGNOSIS

One major pattern of behavior disturbance is a chronic history of serious rule violations; this is the basic concept of a "conduct disorder" as the phrase is generally used in the psychological literature. Although some authors have questioned the validity of conduct disorder as a useful diagnosis (Lewis, Lewis, Unger, & Goldman, 1984), in general it is one of the best-supported DSM diagnoses in both the empirical and clinical literature (Robins, 1991). A habitual pattern of negativistic, oppositional, and defiant behavior that stops short of major rule violations or aggression against people or property is the essential feature of ODD. Conduct problems that do not meet criteria for CD or ODD and appear in response to an identified stress meet the criteria for Adjustment Disorder With Disturbance of Conduct. Bipolar I Disorder, Most Recent Episode Manic and Intermittent Explosive Disorder are rare in children and infrequent in adolescents, but do occur and may present with conduct symptoms. Finally, isolated acts of delinquent or antisocial behavior that do not constitute a pattern of maladjustment can be classified with the V code Child or Adolescent Antisocial Behavior (this is not a mental disorder).

Frequently associated diagnoses or problems that should be considered and ruled in or out when a child presents with apparent CD, ODD, or Disruptive Behavior Disorder NOS include ADHD, Substance Use Disorders, Learning Disorders, Mental Retardation, and abuse and/or neglect. Alternative explanations for conduct problems that should be ruled out include general medical disorders; any recent history of head injury, seizure, or exposure to known neurotoxins; and Psychotic Disorders. The next Application Note summarizes all of these considerations.

Behavior rating scales completed by parents and teachers can be very helpful in establishing the occurrence of disruptive behaviors at frequencies beyond the normal range for given age groups. Differential diagnosis among the various possibilities will require data from either clinical or structured interviews. In addition to the occurrence of major rule violations, another critical feature to be considered in regard to CD is that what is being sought is a *pattern* of behavior, not the occurrence of isolated acts, even if such acts are very serious. In practice, any real questions about a diagnosis of CD are almost always resolved by the passage of time. Youngsters with CD are pathologically unable to control their own behavior, even when they clearly recognize that it is in their own best interest to do so.

If the problems with oppositional behavior have not reached the intensity of major rule violations, then the primary differential diagnosis will be between ODD and Disruptive Behavior Disorder NOS. (A diagnosis of CD precludes the concurrent diagnosis of ODD; the assumption is that all children with CD will also show ODD.) Given the evidence that at least some cases of ODD, but not all, will eventually evolve into CD, the boundaries between these two classifications can be especially difficult to delineate (Biederman et al., 1996). A

APPLICATION NOTE Differential Diagnosis for Disruptive Behavior Problems

Consider:
> CD
> ODD
> Adjustment Disorder With Disturbance of Conduct
> Bipolar I Disorder, Most Recent Episode Manic
> Intermittent Explosive Disorder
> Child or Adolescent Antisocial Behavior (V code)

In addition, consider:
> ADHD
> Substance Use Disorders (adolescents)
> Learning Disorders
> Mental Retardation
> Abuse or neglect

Rule out:
> General medical disorders
> Any recent history of head injury, seizure, or exposure to known neurotoxins
> Psychotic Disorders

case that clearly meets criteria for ODD and includes only one symptom of CD may be best classified as ODD, with supplemental notation of the most serious symptom. A case of ODD with two clear symptoms of CD may be considered for a provisional diagnosis of CD. Consideration of the empirically demonstrated predictive power of individual symptoms can be helpful. For instance, the work of Frick et al. (1994) suggests that fighting and other forms of mild aggression are often associated with ODD.

Despite their high comorbidity, CD, ODD, and Disruptive Behavior Disorder NOS on the one hand and ADHD on the other are conceptually and empirically distinct diagnoses. Given their frequent association, evidence of either type of disorder should prompt a specific review to rule in or rule out the presence of the other.

I would suggest the following heuristic for a school psychologist confronted with a child or adolescent exhibiting disruptive behavior problems. First, does the case present with the essential feature of CD? If CD can be diagnosed, this will take precedence over ODD,

Adjustment Disorder, and Disruptive Behavior Disorder NOS. If the criteria for CD are not present, then I would consider the criteria for ODD. If there is no pattern of either CD or ODD, then I would consider whether the behavior developed in response to psychosocial stress; if so, Adjustment Disorder With Disturbance of Conduct should be diagnosed. Finally, if characteristic features of a Disruptive Behavior Disorder are present but none of the specific diagnoses are justified, a diagnosis of Disruptive Behavior Disorder NOS should be entertained. An evaluation of attention deficit problems, impulsivity, and hyperactivity should accompany these considerations. Given the high comorbidity between Disruptive Behavior Disorders and ADHD, the school psychologist should always consider whether the criteria for ADHD are met when reviewing a case presenting behavior problems.

SPECIFIC BEHAVIOR PATTERNS

Conduct Disorder

The symptom set used to identify Conduct Disorder (CD) in DSM-IV was revised to include two new items the field trials suggested would increase sensitivity to conduct problems in females: staying out late at night without caretaker approval, and intimidating others. The symptoms of CD occur at low base rates among youth (this is consistent with the seriousness/psychopathology of these symptoms). It is therefore not surprising that empirical studies find these symptoms to have high positive predictive power but low negative predictive power. That is, the presence of CD symptoms is highly predictive of other symptoms and of the syndrome, but the absence of a symptom does not predict absence of the disorder (Frick et al., 1994).

The approach to subtyping of CD in DSM-IV is based on age of onset of symptoms. If at least one symptom of CD has been manifested before age 10, the Childhood-Onset Type is identified; if all symptoms develop after age 10, the Adolescent-Onset Type is specified. (An Unspecified Onset option has recently been added, and the three subtypes have received their own specific ICD-9-CM codes; see the following Coding Note.) The Childhood Onset Type is believed to be more strongly associated with aggressive behavior and with risk of later adult Antisocial Personality Disorder. There is evidence for the validity of this approach to subtyping, as well as evidence for the validity of subtyping based on pattern of social affiliation (socialized/group/gang CD vs. unsocialized/undersocialized/isolated CD) or on

CODING NOTE   Coding Changes for Subtypes of CD

The ICD-9-CM is annually reviewed and updated by a federal committee, the ICD-9-CM Coordination and Maintenance Committee. This committee submits proposed changes to the Health Care Financing Administration (HCFA). Following a period of public review and then approval by the director of the HCFA, the final coding changes are published as an Interim Final Notice in the May–June issue of the *Federal Register*. The American Psychiatric Association recently distributed a pamphlet entitled *Coding Changes to DSM-IV Classification* (American Psychiatric Association, 1996a) and published a *DSM-IV Coding Update* (American Psychiatric Association, 1996) to present 23 updated codes affecting DSM-IV diagnostic categories and 7 updated codes from DSM-IV Appendix G ("ICD-9-CM Codes for Selected General Medical Conditions and Medication-Induced Disorders"). One of the categories affected is CD, which was previously coded as 312.8 for all three subtypes (Childhood-Onset Type, Adolescent-Onset Type, and Unspecified Onset). The revised coding identifies each subtype:

312.81   Conduct Disorder, Childhood-Onset Type
312.82   Conduct Disorder, Adolescent-Onset Type
312.89   Conduct Disorder, Unspecified Onset

pattern of aggression (impulsive/reactive/hostile/affective aggression vs. controlled/proactive/instrumental/predatory aggression) (see Christian, Frick, Hill, Tyler, & Frazier, 1997; Vitiello & Stoff, 1997). The superiority of one typology over another has yet to be convincingly demonstrated. Each version of DSM that has considered CD, from DSM-II (American Psychiatric Association, 1968) onward, has employed a different (but related) subtyping approach.

For clients over the age of 18 years, a diagnosis of Antisocial Personality Disorder preempts a diagnosis of CD. Because a history of CD is required for the diagnosis of Antisocial Personality Disorder, all clients who meet the criteria for the latter have met the criteria for CD in the past and will presumably continue to meet it. Rather than artificially generating multiple diagnoses, DSM-IV resolves this situation with the rule that Antisocial Personality Disorder precludes a concurrent diagnosis of CD.

Comorbid diagnoses strongly associated with CD include ADHD, Learning Disorders, and (in adolescence) Substance Use Disorders. Youth with CD tend to use alcohol and other drugs earlier, more often, and more intensely, and to sample a wider range of psychoactive substances. Highly dangerous forms of substance use, such as inhalant use, have been found to be associated with CD (McGarvey, Canterbury, & Waite, 1996). Other comorbid diagnoses seen with some frequency include Mood Disorders, Anxiety Disorders, and Borderline Intellectual Functioning (not a mental disorder). Nonspecific attention problems, lower tested intelligence in the normal range, and impulsivity are also commonly seen traits. A specific risk associated with CD in an adolescent females is the risk of pregnancy and single motherhood (Zoccolillo, Meyers, & Assiter, 1997), which can have multiple short- and long-range implications for both the new mother and her child. In a child or adolescent with CD, a careful review of other areas of adjustment requiring impulse control is warranted.

Assessment of comorbidity in cases of CD is clinically useful, because this appears to be one variable associated with course and prognosis for adult outcome. In general, young people with two identifiable disorders have more difficulty than those with only one; those with three disorders face more challenges than those with two; and so on. Lynam (1996) has argued on the basis of his research that the child or adolescent with comorbid ADHD or ADHD-like problems *and* CD or conduct problems is at much greater risk for chronic offending into adulthood and eventual diagnosis of psychopathy than the youth with only one of these serious behavior problems. My own experience has been CD and Substance Use Disorders in adolescents how a potent negative synergy: Each markedly exacerbates the maladjustment associated with the other pattern of problems. Similar destructive interactions can be observed in the young person who is burdened with both conduct problems and a Learning Disorder. Careful assessment of comorbid problems, even if these do not reach diagnostic criteria, can yield a much fuller picture of the child's or adolescent's struggles in the world and can allow for better anticipation of future complications.

Oppositional Defiant Disorder

ODD as defined by DSM-IV identifies a more seriously maladjusted group of children than did the criterion set of DSM-III-R (Angold & Costello, 1996). This was one of the intentions of the committee, in order to reduce the number of false-positive diagnoses; however, it also further blurs the distinction between ODD and CD, and excludes from diagnosis a number of children with very problematic behaviors that adversely affect their school, community, and/or home adjustment. Many of these children, as well as some of the similar mild cases of ADHD excluded under the new pervasive manifestation requirement (see below), will probably end up diagnosed with the new Disruptive Behavior Disorder NOS category.

The evidence at this time suggests that not all children with ODD go on to develop the more serious CD. Nevertheless, children with a history of ODD, especially if treatment effects are limited, should be occasionally reconsidered for possible exacerbation of the intensity and quality of their acting-out behavior. A subset of children who have been appropriately classified as ODD *will* eventually develop CD. Reviews of the available empirical studies suggest that ODD and CD are distinct patterns but are related: ODD tends to show an earlier onset than CD; a history of ODD is almost universal in children who are diagnosed with CD (but, again, not all children with ODD progress to having CD); and familiar correlates of ODD and CD are reported to be similar, with CD showing a greater density of these variables (Lahey, Loeber, Quay, Frick, & Grimm, 1992; Loeber, Lahey, & Thomas, 1991). Identifying the most optimal sets of symptoms both to establish ODD and CD, and to discriminate between them, remains a challenge. The CD symptom pertaining to frequent bullying, threatening, or intimidating of others, for instance, may actually be more closely associated with ODD than with CD (Burns, Walsh, Owen, & Snell, 1997). In "borderline" cases where this is one of the deciding symptoms, extra caution in reviewing the entire clinical picture is warranted.

Disruptive Behavior Disorder Not Otherwise Specified

Disruptive Behavior Disorder NOS is a new diagnostic category in DSM-IV and should increase the examiners' flexibility in dealing with classification problems. Potential uses of this category include cases where young people present with evidence of acting out but the available data only support two symptoms of CD (at least three are required for diagnosis), or where the pattern of difficulties cannot be documented over the required 6-month period. Given the disturbing tendencies of conduct problems to persist and grow worse over time, examiners can expect that many cases assigned an initial diagnosis of Disruptive Behavior Disorder NOS will qialify for a more specific diagnosis (CD or ODD) as subsequent data are collected.

Intermittent Explosive Disorder

Within the chapter on Impulse-Control Disorders Not Elsewhere Classified DSM-IV includes the classification Intermittent Explosive Disorder to identify discrete episodes of loss of control of aggression that are not typical of an individual's usual adjustment. The behavior in question is generally quite intense, leading to physical assault or destruction of property; and it is judged to be out of proportion to any provocation that occurred. Of critical importance is that the behavior stands in contrast to the client's normal patterns of adjustment or maladjustment—the aggression is not typical of this young person. Other Mental Disorders that could explain extreme aggression (Conduct Disorder, ADHD, a Manic Episode, a Psychotic Disorder, Borderline or Antisocial Personality Disorders) take precedence over Intermittent Explosive Disorder and would have to be ruled out before this diagnosis would be appropriate. Similarly, any substance use or medical condition that could account for unusual aggressiveness would need to be excluded. There may be suspicious physical conditions or events, a history of mild head injury, for example, that cannot be conclusively linked to the acute aggressive episodes. But if a casual association between such a neurological event or illness could be meaningfully argued, the diagnosis of Intermittent Explosive Disorder would not be made. The diagnosis, in the example of a brain injury causing aggressive acting out, would be Personality Change Due to Head Trauma, Aggressive Type. As this demonstrates, the exclusion of alternative explantions is critical to the diagnosis of Intermittent Explosive Disorder.

I would recommend that examiners use due caution in applying this classification to children or adolescents. It should not be used as a "catchall" for cases of violence that are not immediately understood. I have found several instances in which a more careful review of a youth's actual substance use resolved the question of posssible Intermittent Explosive Disorder clearly in the negative. There are, nevertheless, instances in which this would be the most appropriate diagnosis, and it should be considered in cases where "unusual aggressive outbursts" are reported. Additionally, a thorough medical evaluation of the child would be prudent, given the association of explosive behavior with a number of neurological disorders and the need to exclude these as explanations.

Adjustment Disorder With Disturbance of Conduct

An Adjustment Disorder With Disturbance of Conduct diagnosis requires two initial features: (1) identification of an apparent functional relationship between identified situational stress and the development of behavior problems (in this case, problems of conduct); and (2) a symptom picture of conduct problems that does not meet criteria for any specific Axis I syndrome or disorder. Failure to meet either of these conditions invalidates this diagnosis. An additional consideration is that this diagnosis is usually only maintained for a limited period of time. In DSM-III and DSM-III-R, a diagnosis of Adjustment Disorder was only valid for 6 months in children and adults; this was inconsistent with clinical experience and the empirical literature (Newcorn & Strain, 1992). DSM-IV is much less rigid than previous editions in the duration exclusion of Adjustment Disorder diagnoses, but the conceptualization clearly remains that of a transient disorder. Prolonged problems should prompt reconsideration of the most appropriate diagnosis. If the behavior problems persist more than 6 months after termination of the precipitating stressor, the diagnosis is no longer appropriate.

Attention-Deficit/Hyperactivity Disorder

Among the diagnostic and treatment questions most frequently presented to school psychologists are those concerning problems with overactivity, impulsivity, and distractibility which are often diagnosed as ADHD. Multiple questions and controversies surround this topic, but the conceptualization of ADHD within DSM-IV appears to have significant relevance for educational settings (McBurnett, Lahey, & Pfiffner, 1993; see the next IDEA Note).

Within DSM-IV, the diagnosis of ADHD focuses on clinical identification of one or both of two problem syndromes inattention and hyperactivity–impulsivity adversely affecting a child's adjustment in at least two major settings. The change from the single-setting formulation of DSM-III-R to the two setting ("pervasive") formulation of DSM-IV is a significant revision aimed expressly at addressing a perceived overdiagnosis of "borderline" cases (excessive false-positive diagnostic errors). This changes also increases the congruence between DSM-IV and ICD-9-CM and ICD-10, which define ADHD in terms of multiple affected settings. The ultimate effect is to reduce the population of children formally identified as having ADHD, to increase the average severity of impairment of the population of children diagnosed with ADHD, and to increase the homogeneity of this population. It is clear that some children who could have been clearly diagnosed with ADHD in DSM-III-R would not qualify for the diagnosis in DSM-IV (but possibly would qualify for ADHD NOS).

The diagnosis of ADHD has two subtypes (as well as a Combined Type): Predominantly Inattentive Type and Predominantly Hyperactive–Impulsive Type. The validity of this distinction appears to be well supported both clinically and empirically (Lahey, Schaughency, Hynd,

IDEA NOTE   ADHD and IDEA

Despite discussion of its possible inclusion, ADHD was not added to the list of qualifying conditions in the definition of "children with disabilities" in the 1990 revision that transformed Part B of the Education of the Handicapped Act (P.L. 94-142) into IDEA (P.L. 101-476). It was the position of the U.S. Department of Education that ADHD did not need to be added as a separate disability, because children who need special services may be eligibile for such services under the "other health impaired" category if their attention deficits handicap their educational performance (Davila, Williams, & MacDonald, 1991, pp. 2–3). Also, the symptoms of ADHD may meet the eligibility criteria for other mandated categories—"specific learning disability" or "seriously emotionally disturbed" (Davila et al., Williams, & MacDonald, 1991, p. 3). Thus, if the symptoms of ADHD impair children's learning, the children may qualify for special education and/or other services under several existing categories. The diagnosis of ADHD per se, however, does not qualify a child for inclusion under the provisions of IDEA (Davila et al., 1991, p. 4); only if the symptoms are severe enough for the child to meet the definition of "handicapped person" will he or she be eligible for services (Davila et al., 1991, 5). It is interesting to consider that the same argument could have been made about either "autism" or "traumatic brain injury," but that these conditions were added to the list of qualifying conditions in IDEA.

Carlson & Nievas, 1987; Lahey, Schaughency, Strauss, & Frame, 1984). If the child meets the criteria for both Predominantly Inattentive Type and Predominantly Hyperactive–Impulsive Type, then the diagnosis of Combined Type is made. In evaluating possible attention deficits without hyperactivity (ADHD, Inattentive Type), it is worth considering two symptoms that are not included in the DSM-IV criterion list: "often drowsy and sluggish" and "often daydreams." Both have very high positive predictive power (actually better than many of the symptoms on the criterion list), but they have low negative predictive power; in other words, their absence is of little informative value (Frick et al, 1994). With regard to the Predominantly Hyperactive–Impulsive Type, the symptoms of running around and climbing excessively, and of acting as if driven by a motor, have consistently shown high predictive value. A symptom used in DSM-III-R but dropped from DSM-IV for this pattern—engaging in physically risky activities without reflection—has high positive predictive power but low negative predictive power.

Evidence of this characteristic strongly suggests Predominantly Hyperactive–Impulsive ADHD, but its absence does not connote the absence of ADHD (Frick et al., 1994). In contrast, the symptoms of inattention may be relatively nonspecific symptoms of child behavior disorder (Halperin, Matier, Bedi, Sharma, & Newcorn, 1992) and are of little help in differentiating among ADHD, the Disruptive Behavior Disorders, Mood Disorders, Anxiety Disorders, and Psychotic Disorders.

The changes in formulation of ADHD in DSM-IV appear to have met the goals of reducing the heterogeneity of the population diagnosed with this disorder, providing specific criteria for the Predominantly Inattentive Type that are supported by empirical research, and identifying more impaired girls and preschool children (Lahey et al., 1994). The return to a differentiation between distractible–inattentive and hyperactive–impulsive syndromes is well supported (Sabatino & Vance, 1994) and appears to have been well received within school systems (Erk, 1995; Gaub & Carlson, 1997). However, questions regarding associated risks and relationships of the ADHD subtypes remain. Power and DuPaul (1996b) wonder whether the Predominantly Hyperactive–Impulsive Type may not functionally operate to identify younger children who are at risk for eventually "exhibit[ing] the full symptomatic picture of the Combined type" (p. 291).

Efforts certainly have been directed at making the category of ADHD useful and acceptable within a school setting (McBurnett et al., 1993). Despite these accomplishments, concerns about the high heterogeneity of diagnosed populations remain (Baumgaertel, Wolraich, & Dietrich, 1995). Disagreement also persists regarding the role of clinical judgment, possible bias, and the role of developmentally adjusted norms in the diagnosis of ADHD (Power & DuPaul, 1996b). DSM-IV does not address how the clinical information upon which to base a diagnosis of ADHD is to be gathered. Some authorities strongly recommend the use of behavior rating scales with age- and gender-appropriate norms (e.g., Barkley, 1990, 1991b). I find such instruments invaluable in the assessment of ADHD and related disorders. DSM-IV does specify that the frequency and intensity of symptoms must be "maladaptive and *inconsistent with developmental level*" (p. 83; emphasis added). The text points out diagnostic difficulties associated with age-appropriate behaviors in active children, as well as with the need to consider the behaviors from the reference point of the child's mental age in children with Mental Retardation. Although the examiner is free to make these comparisons in whatever manner seems appropriate, the use of age-graded norms certainly facilitates decision making. It is necessary to remember, however, that behavioral rating scales and decision rules can inform the examiner but do not reduce his or her ultimate responsibility. Behavior rating scales are not without their own problems, especially in terms of possible subcultural differences among populations of youth (Reid, 1995). The position of DSM-IV, though a source of consternation to some, is clear on this point: It is the clinical judgment of the professional examiner that establishes the presence of symptoms to support a diagnosis of ADHD (or, indeed, of any mental disorder or other condition).

Another continuing issue of contention regarding diagnosis of ADHD concerns the age-of-onset criterion. DSM-IV requires that at least "some" symptoms of ADHD must have been present and caused impairment before the child reached the age of 7 years. This criterion is consistent with DSM-III and DSM-III-R, which required onset of ADD and ADHD, respectively, before age 7; there was no age-of-onset expectation specified for the Hyperkinetic Reaction of Childhood (or Adolescence) of DSM-II. Note that this requirement is not that the child met full criteria for a diagnosis of ADHD prior to age 7—only that some characteristics were evident and had discernible negative repercussions in the child's life prior to this age. For most child clinical presentations of ADHD, this criterion is of minor significance. In the majority of cases, ADHD manifests itself early in children's development and is readily commented upon by various caretakers.

The age-of-onset criterion has become more of an issue with the increased appreciation of attention problems in adults, some of whom were not diagnosed previously during childhood. This may be especially problematic for children and adolescents with ADHD, Predominantly Inattentive Type (Applegate et al., 1997). Barkley and Biederman (1997) have argued that a set age-of-onset criterion is not well supported by scientific data and creates practical problems in the assessment of adolescents and adults being evaluated for ADHD. In particular, the accuracy of retrospective accounts by caretakers (some of which are given years from the time of interest) may be suspect, even when they involve rather dramatic behavioral symptoms. Barkley and Biederman (1997) suggest that the age-of-onset criterion should be dropped or significantly broadened. For the present, however, the criterion is in place and should be considered as a necessary element of classification. The ADHD NOS classification will be correct for the unusual case of a child or adolescent who currently meets symptomatic criteria for ADHD but for whom an onset of at least some symptoms causing impairment prior to age 7 cannot be established.

Frequent comorbid problems with ADHD include Learning Disorders, the Disruptive Behavior Disorders (CD, ODD, and Disruptive Behavior Disorder NOS), Mood Disorders, and (in adolescents) Substance Use Disorders. The various links between ADHD and Substance Use Disorders and substance use constitute a topic of contining investigation and concern. Lynskey and Fergusson's (1995) analysis of a large cohort of New Zealand children suggested that the association between attention deficits and later substance use was mediated almost entirely by the association between attention problems and conduct problems. Even if this conclusion is supported by subsequent work, the association between ADHD and conduct problems is strong enough to warrant careful monitoring of substance use in youth identified with ADHD.

The best understanding of the relationship between ADHD and Bipolar Disorder continues to be a challenge for practitioners and investigators. In some cases, ADHD precedes by years the development of manic symptoms and may be an early developmental manifestation of Bipolar I Disorder. In other cases, ADHD and Bipolar I Disorder seem to be distinct but comorbid conditions. Faraone, Biederman, Mennin, Wozniak, and Spencer (1997), who studied a large clinical sample, concluded that comorbid DSM-III-R ADHD and Bipolar Disorder in children was familially distinct from other patterns of ADHD and might reflect what had been called "childhood-onset Bipolar Disorder" in the previous literature. At this time, a reasonable recommendation would be for the school psychologist to maintain a sensitivity to possible signs of mania in children being evaluated for ADHD.

Although the clinical picture of ADHD may change, a high percentage of cases continue to manifest clinically meaningful symptoms into adulthood, with great personal morbidity in respect to academic achievement, social adjustment, occupational success, and individual accomplishment. Periodic reevaluations with respect to the current symptom pattern of ADHD, possible comorbid problems, and functional impact on the child's or adolescent's development and adjustment would appear necessary.

As noted above, the age-of-onset requirement for the DSM-IV diagnosis of ADHD is a major consideration, given the current popularity of and/or concern regarding this diagnosis in adolescents and adults. An appearance of ADHD-like symptoms in an adult or adolescent without a history of similar problems going back to early childhood may be more consistent with other DSM-IV diagnoses (e.g., Major Depressive Disorder, Bipolar I Disorder, Adjustment Disorder, Anxiety Disorders, and Cognitive Disorder NOS), or with some General

Medical Conditions (neurological and systemic diseases). If alternative explanations are ruled out, the residual diagnosis of ADHD NOS may be considered.

Children who meet criteria for ADHD, especially the Predominantly Hyperactive–Impulsive and Combined Types, should be considered with respect to ODD. I have observed a high rate of concordance between these two problems, consistent with rates often reported in the literature (Atkins, McKay, Talbott, & Arvanitis, 1996; Barkley, 1990). CD shows strong comorbidity with ADHD (Abikoff & Klein, 1992), as do Substance Use Disorders as the child grows into adolescence. Biederman (1991) has argued that the heterogeneity of ADHD could be meaningfully reduced by considering the presence or absence of aggression as an important subtyping factor. At least some of the negative prognostic associations reported for ADHD may be mediated more by aggression than by ADHD symptoms (Hinshaw, 1992), and aggression can be used as a meaningful basis for distinguishing among children with ADHD (Roberts, 1990).

Learning Disorders also show a high association with ADHD (Hinshaw, 1992), perhaps especially with the Predominantly Inattentive Type (August & Garfinkel, 1989). Halperin et al. (1990) have suggested a cognitive versus behavioral subtyping of ADHD. A careful screening for learning problems is always wise in children and adolescents diagnosed with ADHD. Tested intelligence may be an important prognostic factor in children with ADHD (Aman, Pejeau, Osborne, Rojahn, & Handen, 1996). Data concerning a child's mental ability can be noted on Axis II, regardless of whether a codable condition exists.

Additional comorbid conditions frequently seen in children with ADHD are Mood Disorders and Anxiety Disorders. A DSM-III-R Anxiety Disorder has been reported to occur in up to 30 percent of children diagnosed with ADHD, and DSM-III-R Major Depression has been noted to co-occur with ADHD at the same rate (Barkley, 1991a). Biederman (1991) has also suggested subtyping ADHD on the basis of additional diagnoses of emotional problems. In general, as noted earlier, the prognosis for two identified problems is worse than the prognosis for one, and the prognosis for three problems is worse than the likely outcome for two.

Attention-Deficit/Hyperactivity Disorder Not Otherwise Specified

ADHD NOS provides for the diagnosis of behavior disorders that show the essential feature of ADHD ("a persistent pattern of inattention and/or hyperactivity–impulsivity that is more frequent and severe than is typically observed in individuals of a comparable level of development," p. 78), but that do not meet full criteria for ADHD. For instance, consider a child who shows 5 symptoms from the Predominantly Inattentive Type criterion list and 5 symptoms from the Predominantly Hyperactive–Impulsive Type list. Even though this child has 10 symptoms of ADHD, he or she does not show the requisite 6 from one group or the other. The appropriate diagnosis in this case is ADHD NOS. In all likelihood, further assessment of this child will turn up another symptom from one list or the other, at which time the diagnosis can be changed to the more specific type of ADHD. The examiner should note that this case is different from that of a child who at one time fully met criteria for one of the three specific patterns of ADHD (Combined, Predominantly Inattentive, or Predominantly Hyperactive–Impulsive), has shown remission of some (but not all) of the symptoms over time, and continues to show clinical impairment and/or distress secondary to the remaining symptoms of ADHD. This second child should be diagnosed as having ADHD, [Name of Type], In Partial Remission.

It may also be possible to use the ADHD NOS category for individuals with an onset of symptoms after the age of 7. However, my experience is that this is a very unusual development, and I would recommend great caution in making this application. As ADHD has achieved popularity and familiarity in general publications, it has been seized upon by some individuals looking for an explanation of their difficulties. Attention problems are not unique to ADHD, and in fact are common in many mental disorders—as are problems with productivity, difficulties in interpersonal relationships, and impulsivity. Only when the problems occur within the context of specific behavioral syndromes, cause impairment across at least two settings, and arise early in life does the diagnosis of ADHD usually apply.

◆

See IDEA 1977 Note: Disruptive Behavior Disorders and IDEA 1997, in 2002 Updates, pages 234–235.

CHAPTER 5

♦♦♦

Emotional Symptoms (Internalizing Problems)

♦

ANXIETY PROBLEMS

Overview

Anxiety is a ubiquitous human experience, and anxiety symptoms are common in children and adolescents as they react to the familial, social, academic, and personal challenges of development. When nervousness, tension, and other anxiety reactions become more intense, prolonged, and disruptive than typical, the possibility of an Anxiety Disorder or other anxiety-based mental disorder presents itself. Doll's (1996) review of epidemiological studies found DSM-III and DSM-III-R Anxiety Disorders to be among the most frequently diagnosed patterns of disturbance in school children. Our understanding of anxiety problems in young people has advanced appreciably since Miller et al.'s (1974) seminal discussion, but many remaining issues and controversies continue to make this an often perplexing topic. Certain difficulties derive from the nature of the anxiety response itself, while others reflect the specific developmental differences between anxiety problems in adults and those in children and adolescents (Birmaher et al., 1997).

The concept of anxiety has been both invaluable and frustrating to many investigators and therapists. Anxiety is a multifaceted construct that can be considered and measured from several perspectives—physiological, behavioral, cognitive, and phenomenological.

Our understanding of the biological basis of anxiety has grown tremendously over the past few decades, with fuller knowledge of the neurological and neurohormonal systems involved in the experience of tension, anxiety, fear, and panic. Multiple physical symptoms are often readily apparent in anxiety reactions: Increased striated muscle tension, muscle tremor, changes in perspiration and salivation, increased heart rate, increased blood pressure, temperature changes in the extremities, shifts in stomach acidity and gastric activity, perceptual phenomena associated with increased facial muscle tension, and changes in brain activity have all been investigated. In addition to expanding our understanding of what anxiety is, these physical changes have provided different means of assessing anxiety. Many different physical measures of tension have been developed for laboratory investigations. A potentially significant development was the recognition that various physiological measures of anxiety do not perfectly covary and that a great deal of individual variability exists in different people's responsiveness along different biological channels when presented with anxiety-evoking stimuli. Although our present diagnostic categories remain based on historically recognized patterns of subjectively reported experiences and observed behavioral characteristics, there is a very real possibility that future diagnostic formulations may be based on different biological systems mediating anxiety responses.

Behavioral or motoric aspects of anxiety involve the typical avoidance or escape behavior seen when an individual is confronted with cues evoking high levels of fear. Intense anxiety is usually an aversive experience, and reduction of fear typically functions as a negative reinforcer. For example, children confronted with a frightening dog next door will run away to escape from it; later they will avoid going into that yard to prevent another encounter with the beast. Successful escape and avoidance are strengthened by the arousal reduction they produce or maintain. A common conceptual formulation of anxiety problems is that they are exaggerated anxiety control responses that are no long functional. Although escape from actual danger (either physical danger or a threat to self-esteem) is usually adaptive, excessive reactions to overestimated threats tend to cause too much distress or limit effective coping. Early in my career, I evaluated an adolescent with a snake phobia, who had responded to his roommate's throwing a rubber snake at him by scrambling out his second-floor bedroom window. He risked serious physical harm, motivated by a fear he knew to be unrealistic.

The cognitive aspects of anxiety reflect the disruption of higher mental processes seen with elevated tension and arousal. Thinking, abstract reasoning, planning, problem solving, and effective recall are all interfered with by high anxiety. When our students tell us they really know more than their test scores indicate, there is often a core of truth in their rationalization. Anxiety interferes with cognitive processing. Although many adolescents may maintain that they perform best (or can only perform) under pressure, the weight of the evidence is against this position.

Finally, there is the phenomenological or subjective experience of anxiety that is so familiar to most of us. There is a sense of dread, despair, and impending doom that we cannot control. We may experience sensations of suffocation; fears of impending death; anticipation of unarticulated catastrophe; and loss of control over our breath, swallowing, speech, and coordination. Anxiety is part of human life, and most of us are more familiar than we would care to be with the private experience of this most human emotion. Adolescents, like adults, can easily learn to capture this subjective experience with various reporting devices such as "Subjective Units of Disturbance" (SUDs; Wolpe, 1990), 100-millimeter lines, and other rating scales. Children can usually learn to use age-appropriate analogue reporting methods, such as "fear thermometers."

These aspects of anxiety are not rigidly compartmentalized, but fade into each other. For instance, when a student "forgets" about a forthcoming test that he or she has been very worried about, is this avoidance a cognitive or a behavioral manifestation? More important than worrying about abstract boundaries is the recognition that anxiety is a complex response with multiple manifestations (i.e., symptoms). Anxiety symptoms occur as part of many psychiatric disorders. Anxiety symptoms are common in depression and other Mood Disorders, as well as in Somatoform and Dissociative Disorders, in some Sleep Disorders, and in Substance Use Disorders. In fact, in most of the disorders classified in DSM-IV, anxiety symptoms may sometimes occur. But when the anxiety symptoms are the primary manifestations of difficulty, we can conceptualize the problem as a potential Anxiety Disorder (or other anxiety-based mental disorder) and begin looking for characteristic patterns of symptoms—anxiety syndromes such as Panic Attacks or Agoraphobia, and other recognized clinical pictures such as phobias, obsessive–compulsive reactions, or posttraumatic stress reactions. The organizing distinction among "symptoms," "syndromes," and "disorders" is very helpful here. Anxiety symptoms are common in all children at different times and circumstances. Anxiety syndromes, clusters of symptoms covarying together, occur less commonly and for varying period of duration. When an anxiety syndrome persists for some minimal duration and causes either significant personal distress or functional impairment, the essential requirements for an Anxiety Disorder (or other disorder centering around anxiety) are met.

The "Anxiety Disorders" chapter of DSM-IV brings together most of the syndromes and disorders in this classification system where anxiety symptoms are the primary clinical concern. For children and adolescents, the principal additional categories are Separation Anxiety Disorder, Adjustment Disorder with Anxiety, and Avoidant Personality Disorder. (I discuss Avoidant Personality Disorder in this chapter in connection with the differential diagnosis of Social Phobia; it is discussed further in its own right in Chapter 10.) The next IDEA Note sets forth how these disorders relate to eligibility for services under IDEA.

IDEA NOTE   Anxiety-Related Mental Disorders and IDEA

A diagnosis of an Anxiety Disorder (or other mental disorder centering around anxiety) can form the basis of qualifying a child for special services under the "seriously emotionally disturbed" category of IDEA. One of the identified conditions indicating "seriously emotionally disturbed" is a "tendency to develop physical symptoms or fears associated with personal or school problems" that persists "over a period of time" and "adversely affects educational performance" (U.S. Department of Health, Education and Welfare, 1977, p. 42478). Severe anxiety symptoms can easily be construed as falling within this condition. Another identified condition is "an inability to build or maintain satisfactory relationships with peers and teachers," which can be a symptom associated with anxiety problems in children and adolescents. Documentation of the functional impairment in academic or social adjustment caused by the anxiety problem will be important. The information on Axis IV (Psychosocial and Environmental Problems) and Axis V (Global Assessment of Functioning) may also be important in establishing eligibility for services under IDEA.

The IDEA requirement that the qualifying condition must have a negative impact on educational performance opens the possibility of conundrums in the application of the IDEA system versus the DSM system. It is possible that a child or adolescent might be miserable and show significant social maladjustment but maintain acceptable school performance. This young person, even though manifesting a severe Anxiety Disorder or other related disorder, might not be eligible for services under IDEA. Much more typical, however, is obvious impairment in academic achievement associated with severe anxiety symptoms.

One complication of evaluating Anxiety Disorders and other anxiety problems, especially in children, is that many of the manifestations may be largely in the nature of private experience. Children may be acutely distressed by their fear, worry, and tension; however, unless they report this, act it out in behavioral avoidance/escape, or exhibit a clearly disrupted level of performance in academic or everyday tasks, teachers, parents, or other caretakers may remain unaware of the children's suffering. The difficulties inherent in evaluating private experiences, especially in younger children, necessitate that examiners aggressively explore reports or behaviors suggesting anxiety problems in children and make use of multiple sources of data. Indications from the young persons themselves of problems with anxiety should probably be weighted more heavily than negative reports from caretakers (Cantwell et al., 1997). While remaining cognizant of the reality that fears and even extreme fears are common and usually transient in children, a school psychologist also needs to be sensitive to indications that anxiety phenomena are enduring in a child's life; are causing a great deal of unhappiness; or are contributing to failures in expected personal, social, or academic development. My impression is that anxiety problems are underdiagnosed in school-age children. Adults often fail to recognize there problems or misattribute them to the "normal" vicissitudes of growing up.

Specific Anxiety Patterns

As would be expected, DSM-IV approaches Anxiety Disorders (and other related disorders) by identifying a variety of specific symptom groupings that have been recognized in clinical practice. The broad heuristic for the evaluator is, first, the recognition that many or most of a child's or adolescent's problems can be conceptualized as anxiety difficulties; second, the exclusion of more pervasive problems for which anxiety can be an associated symptom (general medical conditions, Psychotic Disorders, Mood Disorders); and, third, the identification of the specific pattern or patterns of symptoms most characteristic of the young person's problems. The issue of a more pervasive disorder's preempting the diagnosis of less global disorders is very important in the assessment and diagnosis of Anxiety Disorders. Anxiety as a symptom is common in many emotional and behavioral disorders; only when it is the core of the difficulty is an Anxiety Disorder diagnosed. An Anxiety Disorder can be diagnosed concurrently with a Mood Disorder such as Major Depressive Disorder (MDD), but only when there is evidence that the Anxiety Disorder is a separate problem. For instance, if the child has a history of a clinical Phobia for several years and (while this problem continues) then develops MDD, both diagnoses should be made. This example illustrates the basic situation of diagnosing two disorders where one is an associated symptom of the other: In this case, there is evidence of independent occurrence of the two dysfunctions.

Syndromes

The "Anxiety Disorders" chapter of DSM-IV begins by defining two syndromes that are referred to in several specific diagnoses—the often related patterns of Panic Attack and Agoraphobia.

PANIC ATTACK

A Panic Attack is an episode of intense fear, physiological arousal, and (often) frantic escape behavior, occurring during a discrete period of time (i.e., peaking within 10 minutes). Panic Attacks are sufficiently distinct from normal experience and noxious in character that adult clients usually give relatively clear and reliable accounts of their occurrence. Panic Attacks in children have received some discussion in the literature, but little is clear. It is not certain how frequent this experience is prior to adolescence, or even whether it occurs at all prior to puberty (Bernstein & Borchardt, 1991). A recent study by Biederman et al. (1997) suggests that Panic Disorder and Agoraphobia may occur with some frequency in clinical populations, but may not be easily recognized. Research on Panic Attacks in both clinical (Kearney, Albano, Eisen, Allan & Barlow, 1997) and nonclinical (Hayward et al., 1997) populations of youth are beginning to provide a more empirical foundation of knowledge on this subject.

AGORAPHOBIA

Agoraphobia is a frequently seen fear syndrome in adult clinical settings, but it appears to be infrequent in children and adolescents. A commonly offered model of Agoraphobia sees it as usually, but not inevitably, associated with a history of cued or uncued Panic Attacks; Agoraphobia is an acute fear of being in circumstances where the person may be unable to escape or get help if the need arises. Agoraphobia is thought of as a "fear of fear," or catastrophic misinterpretation of physiological cues of increasing tension. Although this view is very appealing, it may not be consistent with the empirical data on the relative prevalence of Panic Attacks and Agoraphobia and their respective ages of onset (Biederman et al., 1997). Many empirical and theoretical questions remain to be resolved regarding these two syndromes.

Although Panic Attacks and Agoraphobia and the several diagnoses built around them (Panic Disorder With Agoraphobia, Panic Disorder Without Agoraphobia, and Agoraphobia Without History of Panic Disorder) may be very useful in conceptualizing adult anxiety problems, in my experience they have limited application to juvenile situations. The remaining Anxiety Disorders are relatively frequent in children and adolescents. In addition, one of the Disorders Usually First Diagnosed in Infancy, Childhood, or Adolescence is a significant anxiety problem in children, and one of the Adjustment Disorder diagnoses focuses on anxiety symptoms.

Anxiety Disorders

COMORBIDITY

A good heuristic rule to keep in mind with respect to Anxiety Disorders is that comorbidity tends to be the rule rather than the exception. Comorbid diagnoses of depressive disorders, Attention-Deficit/ Hyperactivity Disorder (ADHD), and other Anxiety Disorders are common. The frequently reported high correlations between specific Anxiety Disorders raise serious questions about the ultimate utility and validity of the DSM-IV approach to categorizing anxiety problems. The practical implications are that evidence of an Anxiety Disorder in a child or adolescent should prompt a careful review for possible evidence of other Anxiety Disorders, as well as a review of symptoms of Mood Disorders and ADHD. In adolescents, a careful evaluation of alcohol and other substance use should also be made.

SPECIFIC PHOBIA

Fears are common in children, and even intense fears occur with some frequency (Milne et al., 1995). By contrast, a "phobia" has been defined as a "special form of fear" that is excessive, maladaptive, persistent, and (in the case of children) "not age or state specific" (Marks, 1969, quoted in Miller et al., 1974, p. 90). Mild fears are common and usually transient; severe fears are more likely to continue over time; and phobias tend to be stable without systematic intervention. The intensity and predictability of the anxiety reaction to the identified phobic stimulus usually make diagnosis fairly straightforward. Phobia like elements make up part of the clinical picture of Obsessive–

Compulsive Disorder (OCD) and Posttraumatic Stress Disorder (PTSD), as well as of Specific Phobias and Social Phobia.

More so than the other Anxiety Disorders, Specific Phobias—intense, stable fears of discrete situations or objects—can and do occur in isolation from other anxiety or depressive difficulties. Phobias involving blood or injury, for instance, have usually been reported without significant rates of comorbidities (Marks, 1988). If there is a fear of phobic intensity, however, the majority of cases will show other extreme fears (Milne et al., 1995). The important element of a Specific Phobia is the exaggerated anxiety response relative to any degree of actual physical or psychological risk present in the situation, which leads to maladaptive responding. Five subtypes of Specific Phobias may be specified in DSM-IV: Animal Type, Natural Environment Type, Blood–Injection–Injury Type, Situational Type, or Other Type.

SOCIAL PHOBIA

When a phobic reaction is elicited by interpersonal stimuli, the diagnosis of Social Phobia is made. Youth with Social Phobia show extreme anxiety in situations where they feel evaluated by others; they fear being embarrassed, humiliated, or thought poorly of by other people. In some cases, this may center around a particular concern (e.g., blushing). One young adolescent I consulted with could barely stand being looked at by others, because of her fear that she would blush and they would laugh at her. Alternatively, the fear may be a general sense of looking "stupid," saying something "dumb," or being found generally lacking in some undefined way. Whereas social anxieties are relatively common in adolescents and adults, Social Phobia can be conceptualized as an extreme point on a dimension of concern about social evaluation. Its onset is usually in adolescence (Herbert, 1995), and without treatment the course is often chronic, with significant personal, social, and vocational impairment. There is frequent comorbidity with other Anxiety Disorders, depression, as well as an increased risk of Substance Abuse (Herbert, 1995). The sex ratio is approximately equal, and adult prevalence estimates are approximately 2% (Herbert, 1995).

The diagnosis of Social Phobia in children and adolescents brings up boundary issues with Avoidant Personality Disorder, which are difficult to resolve within the directives given by DSM-IV. Both diagnoses focus on anxiety symptoms elicited by interpersonal exposure and interaction. The overlap in defining symptoms yields very high comorbidities. Avoidant Personality Disorder occurs in 25–70% of clients diagnosed with Social Phobia; and Social Phobia, can almost always be diagnosed in clients with Avoidant Personality Disorder (Herbert, 1995). These two categories are probably not distinct phenomenological or symptomatic clusters (Francis, Last, & Strauss, 1992). Avoidant Personality Disorder may well represent a more severe manifestation of the same basic pattern reflected in Social Phobia. Given the thorny conceptual issues in using the concept of a Personality Disorder with adolescents and especially children (see Chapter 10), I would recommend that the category of Social Phobia be used when the differential diagnosis is between this category and Avoidant Personality Disorder.

"School phobia" is not a diagnosis available within DSM-IV. Bernstein and Borchardt (1991) suggest that in a high percentage of cases of school refusal separation anxiety is found to be manifested, and that many of these children may meet criteria for Separation Anxiety Disorder (see below). Some children, however, present with a distinct fear of school rather than Separation Anxiety Disorder, and are probably best conceptualized as having a variant of Social Phobia (Last, Francis, Hersen, Kazdin, & Strauss, 1987). Like young people with other anxiety problems, youth with school avoidance or refusal may not acknowledge that their fears are excessive or unreasonable. Symptoms of school avoidance or refusal may also occur in the cluster of conduct problems where they reflect not anxiety but self-indulgence. For treatment planning, the important differential diagnosis is between school avoidance as a manifestation of an Anxiety Disorder and school avoidance as a manifestation of Disruptive Behavior Disorder.

OBSESSIVE–COMPULSIVE DISORDER

OCD has been increasingly acknowledged as more common in children and adolescents than previously believed, although failure to recognize these problems continues (March & Leonard, 1996). Young people with OCD are often sensitive to the negative reactions of others and may carry out their compulsive behaviors in secret. A child or adolescent may come to the attention of the school psychologist because of secondary problems—academic difficulties caused by obsessive concerns and ritualistic behavior, a teacher's concern over frequent requests to be excused to the washroom, or physical signs of excessive washing (Adams, Waas, March, & Smith, 1994). Common obsessions and compulsions reported in child clinical cases by March and Leonard (1996) are shown in Table 5.1. Washing and checking rituals are reported to occur in most child cases at some point in the clinical course (Swedo, Rapoport, Leonard, Lenane & Cheslow, 1989).

TABLE 5.1. Common Obsessions and Compulsions Reported
in Child Cases

Obsessions	Compulsions
Contamination themes	Washing
Harm to self or others	Repeating
Aggressive themes	Checking
Sexual themes	Touching
Scrupulosity/religiosity	Counting
Forbidden thoughts	Ordering/arranging
Symmetry urges	Hoarding
Need to tell, ask, confess	Praying

Note. From March and Leonard (1996). Copyright 1996 by the American
Academy of Child and Adolescent Psychiatry. Reprinted by permission.

Although either intrusive thoughts or ritualistic behaviors will satisfy
the diagnostic requirements, both types of features are usually seen
in clinical cases. The behavior must cause the young person distress,
or take up excessive amounts of time, or interfere with functional
adjustment (school performance, social activities, or important relationships). Children do not need to recognize the illogical nature of
their behavior (they usually do); With Poor Insight may be noted if
there is not some acknowledgment of the excessive and senseless nature of the symptoms.

Other Anxiety Disorders are often seen in children OCD (especially Specific and Social Phobias and Generalized Anxiety Disorder).
Tic Disorders (including Tourette's Disorder) have been found to be
associated with OCD in some families (March & Leonard, 1996; Pauls,
Alsobrook, Goodman, Rasmussen, & Leckman, 1995). Disruptive
Behavior Disorders and Learning Disorders are reported to be common associated problems of children with OCD; "obsessive–compulsive spectrum disorders" (Trichotillomania, Body Dysmorphic Disorder, and habit problems such as nail biting) are said to occur as less
frequent comorbidities (March & Leonard, 1996). In particular, OCD
and Tourette's Disorder appear in at least some instances to be alternative phenotypical expressions of a common genotype (March &
Leonard, 1996). The recent report of an association among OCD,
Tourette's Disorder, and a trait marker of streptococcal infections will
no doubt intensify the search for a possible neurological foundation
for these disorders (Swedo et al., 1997).

OCD and Obsessive–Compulsive Personality Disorder, despite the
similarity of their titles, do not appear to covary at any meaningful
frequency in children or adolescents.

GENERALIZED ANXIETY DISORDER

Generalized Anxiety Disorder (GAD) involves a grouping of anxiety symptoms and worry that occur without specific eliciting stimuli. The individual shows a pervasive and enduring pattern of excessive arousal. This pattern in children was previously labeled Overanxious Disorder of Childhood; only in DSM-IV it has been formally acknowledged that the child, adolescent, and adult manifestations are essentially identical. Excessive worry ("apprehensive expectation") is a defining feature of GAD that is certainly consistent with the clinical literature on children (Strauss, Lease, Last, & Francis, 1988). High comorbidities are reported with other Anxiety Disorders, MDD, and ADHD—a pattern of comorbidity seen for many Anxiety Disorders in children, as noted earlier.

POSTTRAUMATIC STRESS DISORDER

PTSD involves a triad of defining symptoms following exposure to a extremely traumatic stressor. The core symptoms are (1) a recurrent reexperiencing of the stressor, (2) persistent avoidance of reminders of the event and a decrease in general responsiveness ("numbing"), and (3) persistent hyperarousal. Some amount of controversy has surrounded this diagnosis since its introduction in DSM-III, but overall both the clinical experience of practitioners and the empirical literature appear to support its basic validity and utility. Critical concerns about the accurate diagnosis of PTSD center on three issues, which are discussed below: (1) the nature of the stressful event, (2) the defining pattern of symptoms, and (3) the course of the disorder. Important additional topics beyond the scope of this discussion include the possibility of individual differences or premorbid risk factors that may predispose children to develop PTSD, and possible neurological changes underlying PTSD. It is worth noting that PTSD is one of the very few disorders for which DSM-IV specifies etiological circumstances.

The Nature of the Traumatic Stress. DSM-III and DSM-III-R built the category of PTSD around the concept of a psychologically disturbing event that is beyond the range of typical human experience. This notion proved very troublesome in application and was ultimately rejected as unworkable. In its Criterion A for PTSD, DSM-IV replaces this formulation with a specification of a traumatic event that has two defining features: (1) There is exposure to the risk or actuality of death, serious harm, or loss of physical integrity; and (2) the client's reaction includes either intense negative emotion (fear, horror, help-lessness) or (in children) disorganized behavior or agitation. This seems to be a more objective and serviceable conceptualization of the circumstances that can evoke this pattern of maladjustment. March (1993) provides a good review of the Criterion A issue. The common causes of child and adolescent trauma include physical and sexual abuse and maltreatment, community and domestic violence, natural disasters, war, and civil conflicts (Putnam, 1996).

However, it appears clear from the available clinical and empiri-cal literature that the various types of traumatic events just mentioned do not *inevitably* lead to PTSD (McNally, 1993). These highly distress-ing experiences may be sufficient to elicit PTSD, but they are neither necessary nor inexorably sufficient. In the current social climate, it may be worth emphasizing that this is as true of sexual victimization (rape, incest, or other acute or chronic forms of sexual abuse) as of other types of traumatic events; the tendency at present is to assume that sexual abuse invariably results in PTSD, but this is not the case. The topics of risk factors and of possible protective factors (both sub-ject variables and post trauma experiences) are very exciting points of investigation in this area. Suffice it to say here that automatically diagnosing PTSD for any child with a history of sexual abuse (or any other traumatic experience) can would lead to many errors of classi-fication and constitutes a misuse of this category.

The Defining Symptom Pattern. As noted above, the essential symp-tom picture for PTSD involves the manifestation of three elements: reexperiencing of the traumatic event; avoidance of stimuli connected with the trauma and general "numbing"; and heightened arousal. All three of these must represent a change in the individual's typical be-havior. Several specific symptom manifestations can be used to docu-ment each of the three defining elements. All three must be present for the diagnosis to be made. A positive change in DSM-IV is the ex-plicit discussion of how symptoms may be manifested differently in children. Putnam (1996) offers a valuable discussion of developmen-tal features in PTSD symptoms. The general statement of necessary functional impairment is included in the diagnostic criteria. The du-ration of troublesome symptoms must be at least 1 month.

The identified rate of PTSD is closely tied to the diagnostic crite-rion set used, and the changes from DSM-III to DSM-III-R to DSM-IV have had significant effects on the population of children classified with this disorder (Schwarz & Kowalski, 1991). Schwarz and Kowalski have also commented on the effects of different assessment method-ologies (a self-report questionnaire for adults vs. structured interviews for children) on the detection of PTSD symptoms following a traumatic event. Serial assessment of children exposed to a trauma who show subsyndromal symptoms may be helpful in giving the examiner more opportunity to directly observe possible manifestations of avoidance, arousal, or reexperiencing phenomena. This is a particular consideration with very young children, whose diagnosis is complicated by their developmental status. Scheeringa, Zeanah, Drell, and Larrieu (1995) have suggested modifications of the DSM-IV PTSD criteria for use with infants and children younger than 48 months. Although such revisions may be very useful, it will be important to note whether a diagnosis is based on other than the standard set of criteria.

Motta (1995) provides a nice review of PTSD for school psychologist, including a discussion of frequently observed and reported manifestations in a school setting and a review of assessment instruments and structured interviews. Motta very appropriately comments although such instruments can be helpful in eliciting data supporting a diagnosis of PTSD, assessment results are not the definitive standard: "Rather, school mental health personnel often make judgements based on multiple sources of input including data obtained from actual child behavior, oral report, test and questionnaire data, and the reports of those familiar with the child" (1995, p. 70). This statement is very consistent with the philosophy and clinical application of DSM-IV.

Epidemiological studies have found PTSD disturbingly frequent in youth. Giaconia et al. (1995) found that by age 18 more than 6% of a community sample of young people had met criteria for a diagnosis of PTSD at some point in their lives. They also found that partial symptomatology was common and could be very disabling even when full criteria for the diagnosis were not met. Pfefferbaum's review (1997) recommended clinical consideration of partial syndromes for treatment, especially in children where the chronic course of untreated PTSD can disrupt development.

The Course of PTSD. DSM-IV notes that PTSD can occur at any age and that the symptom picture may fluctuate over time. Complete recovery is reported to occur in roughly half of clinical cases within 3 months (p. 426); however, some cases persist stubbornly over years. A troublesome issue in clinical practice is that as the symptom picture improves, either over time or in response to effective treatment, a child may no longer fully meet the criteria for PTSD. This can initially be dealt with by describing the disorder as In Partial Remission, but as the child continues to improve, a decision regarding reclassification will eventually to be called for. DSM-IV does not offer any guidance here. My own practice is to view the reexperiencing of the trauma and/or the suppression of emotional responsiveness ("numbing") as the unique core of this diagnosis, and to maintain the diagnosis as long as either of these is evident in the clinical picture. Avoidance and overarousal are features of several Anxiety Disorders and are not unique to PTSD; thus, the continuation of only these symptoms is not sufficient for me to retain this diagnostic formulation.

Significant comorbidities are reported for other Anxiety Disorders, as well as for MDD, Somatization Disorder, and Substance-Related Disorders. Most clinical cases of PTSD meet criteria for another mental disorder. Substance involvement (alcohol use, as well as illicit and prescription drug use) should be carefully reviewed, especially in chronic cases. A recent study by Deykin and Buka (1997) suggests that there may be important gender differences in patterns of comorbidity between Substance Dependence and PTSD. The female adolescents in this study tended to develop chemical dependency after the establishment of PTSD, possibly to control the emotional distress associated with the stress reaction. In the male adolescents, the Substance Dependence tended to be the primary disorder and to lead to PTSD by causing the teenagers to be exposed to situations in which traumatization was more likely.

ACUTE STRESS DISORDER

The new diagnostic category of Acute Stress Disorder refers to the development of characteristic anxiety and dissociative symptoms within the first month following exposure to a traumatic event qualifying as sufficient for PTSD; the duration (the defining feature) is less than 1 month. The symptom picture is identical to that of PTSD, with two exceptions: (1) The duration is restricted as just noted, and (2) at least three of a group of five dissociative symptoms are required. If maladjustment persists beyond a month, the diagnosis should be changed to another mental disorder (possibly PTSD, possibly some other mental disorder or syndrome).

Acute Stress Disorder and PTSD are mutually exclusive because of the duration elements in the definitions. The addition of a diagnosis of PTSD is a redefinition of the same symptom picture that has been used to document Acute Stress Disorder. The two disorders should not be concurrently diagnosed.

The usefulness of and rationale for requiring dissociative symptoms in addition to the PTSD triad of symptoms is not clear; however, these experiences are common in individuals who have lived through traumatic events, regardless of whether they subsequently develop Acute Stress Disorder or PTSD. Assessment of dissociative symptoms can be problematic. Scales assessing dissociative experiences have been developed for use with children (Helmers, Putnam, & Trickett, 1993) and adolescents (Armstrong, Putnam, Carlson, Libero, & Smith, 1997), and these can be of help in evaluating these symptom areas. (See also "Dissociation Disorders," below.)

It is worth reiterating that neither sexual abuse nor any other traumatic event is necessarily sufficient to elicit the symptoms of PTSD, and by extension does not guarantee development of Acute Stress Disorder. Exposure to an extremely traumatic experience is necessary for these two diagnoses but not sufficient; the diagnoses require the subsequent development of a characteristic symptom pattern.

OTHER ANXIETY DISORDERS

Anxiety Disorders in children and adolescents can develop as a consequence of substance use (Substance-Induced Anxiety Disorder) or a general medical condition (Anxiety Disorder Due to a General Medical Condition). That is, generalized nervousness and tension, fears, Panic Attacks, or obsessive–compulsive symptoms may develop during drug or medication intoxication or withdrawal, as well as in response to illness, injury, or some other physiological influence. Anxiety problems may also develop that do not conform to any of the specific symptom patterns identified (Anxiety Disorder Not Otherwise Specified [NOS]).

Other Anxiety-Related Mental Disorders

SEPARATION ANXIETY DISORDER

Separation Anxiety Disorder is one of the more frequent clinical anxiety presentations in children (Bernstein & Borchardt, 1991) and is one of the few anxiety-related mental disorders for which there is reasonable congruence between child and caretaker reports (Cantwell et al., 1997). It is also the only mental disorder centering around anxiety that is still located in the "Disorders Usually First Diagnosed in Infancy, Childhood, or Adolescence" chapter of DSM-IV. The key feature in the accurate diagnosis of Separation Anxiety Disorder is that a child's separation from his or her primary caretaker serves as the effective stimulus for the intense anxiety reaction. It is seen in situations when the child is being left off at day care or school by the caretaker, or when the child is left home with a babysitter and the caretaker leaves; it is usually quickly relieved by reunion with the caretaker. The child may have problems being apart from the caretaker even within the home (e.g., unwillingness to sleep in his or her own bed). The relationship of this disorder to earlier, developmentally normal fears (fear of strangers, developmentally typical separation anxiety) is of continuing interest.

School avoidance or refusal is reported as a symptom of Separation Anxiety Disorder in the majority of cases (approximately 75%, according to Francis, Last, & Strauss, 1987); however, some care should be taken to evaluate and eliminate the possibility that the fear response is to some stimulus element in the situation (i.e., fear of school or some aspect of school vs. fear of separation from the caretaker). The evaluator should also keep in mind that separation anxiety is common and normal in younger children. Nevertheless, it is very important to evaluate the intensity and quality of a child's separation anxiety experience and its effects upon his or her adjustment. Separation Anxiety Disorder *is* a mental disorder—the anxiety about separation from caretakers is excessive and maladaptive.

ADJUSTMENT DISORDER WITH ANXIETY

Anxiety symptoms can also occur as a reaction to situational stressors in an individual's life. The diagnosis of Adjustment Disorder With Anxiety identifies the development of anxiety symptoms that cause distress or functional impairment (criteria for a mental disorder) and that develop following an identified psychosocial stressor. (Two other subtypes of Adjustment Disorder that involve, or can involve, anxiety symptoms—Adjustment Disorder With Mixed Anxiety and Depressed Mood, and Adjustment Disorder With Mixed Disturbance of Emotions and Conduct—are mentioned later in this chapter.) The relationship of Adjustment Disorders to other Axis I and II disorders is structured by several rules that constrain the use of this diagnostic group. An Adjustment Disorder diagnosis is not made if the problems focused upon can be accounted for by another Axis I mental disorder, even when this disorder appears clearly related etiologically to a psychosocial stressor. For instance, suppose that in apparent response to a bad experience in speaking before his class, a school-age boy shows over the next 6 months a recurrent and persistent fear of public speaking in all situations; responds to required class presentations with evidence of tremor, crying, sweating, and complaints of choking, nausea, and dizziness; attempts to avoid public speaking at almost any cost; and, because of this avoidance, passes up a chance to run for a position as class officer (which he has previously expressed interest in) and reports dreading school (which he has previously enjoyed). The diagnosis in this case should be Social Phobia. This child meets all the criteria for Social Phobia, and therefore this diagnosis is made rather than the diagnosis of Adjustment Disorder With Anxiety.

A diagnosis of Adjustment Disorder is also not made if the problem is seen as a stress-induced exacerbation of an existing Axis I disorder. For instance, if a girl who has previously met criteria for Social Phobia (because of performance anxiety in social situations that caused her clinically significant distress) now begins to manifest active avoidance behavior of group events and parties because she has suffered extreme embarrassment at a social function, the diagnosis of Adjustment Disorder should not be added. The additional symptoms appear to be a further development of the Social Phobia already present.

Furthermore, a diagnosis of Adjustment Disorder is not made if the symptoms persist more than 6 months after the termination of the stressor. As noted in Chapter 4, this is a change in DSM-IV that greatly extends the flexibility of the system and is more consistent with the lives of many clients (Newcorn & Strain, 1992). Previous editions placed rigid time limits on the use of Adjustment Disorder, which ignored not uncommon real-life circumstances: Stressors are sometimes chronic (e.g., a parent's lingering illness or create problems that persist over time (e.g., financial and interpersonal disruption caused by a parent's losing a job). Shifting the criterion from the absolute duration of the disorder to the duration relative to the stressor means that these cases can be more sensibly handled. Adjustment Disorders, however, are viewed as essentially transient events that should eventually resolve. Persistence of the symptoms 6 months beyond the termination of the stressful precipitating events requires a change of the diagnosis to another category—often an NOS diagnosis within the general problem area.

The question of the relationship between Adjustment Disorder With Anxiety and Anxiety Disorder NOS can be problematic for the examiner and is not completely resolved by DSM-IV. Neither of these diagnoses should be made if a child's or adolescent's symptom picture fully meets the criteria for any specific Anxiety Disorder diagnoses. The diagnosis of Adjustment Disorder should be made if there is evidence of anxiety symptoms (as the primary problems) in clear response to an identifiable stressor that have not persisted for over 6 months. The diagnosis of Anxiety Disorder NOS should be made if there is evidence of anxiety symptoms (as the primary problems) that have not been clearly precipitated by an identifiable situational event. The diagnosis of Anxiety Disorder NOS should also be made if the problems have persisted for more than 6 months after the resolution of the stressors. Problematic cases involve symptoms lasting up to 6 months whose relationship to events in the young person's life is questionable. The clear intention of DSM-IV (similar to DSM-III and DSM-III-R) appears to be to constrain the use of Adjustment Disorder diagnoses to be a set of distinct circumstances. Adjustment Disorder was one of the DSM-III-R diagnoses most frequently used with children and adolescents (Newcorn & Strain, 1992), and there continues to be concern about the potential overuse of this category. My recommendation is to use an NOS diagnosis if there is any real question regarding the difficulty's being an (identified) stress-related disturbance.

MOOD PROBLEMS

Overview

The Mood Disorders in DSM-IV are conceptualized as a group of behavioral problems that "have a disturbance in mood as the predominant feature" (p. 317). "Mood" is defined in Appendix C of DSM-IV as "a pervasive and sustained emotion that colors the perception of the world" (p. 768). The key idea is that the mood disturbance is judged to be the primary feature of the individual's problems. This places a considerable responsibility on the examiner both to be sensitive to indications of depression and other affective disturbances in children and adolescents, and to carefully evaluate the complex relationships among different symptom clusters and environmental events in order to arrive at a view of the primary and secondary status of various elements. The nature and manifestation of mood problems in youth have received a great deal of attention over recent decades. The idea of serious affective disturbance as a clinical problem in young people, especially children, has been difficult for some investigators to accept, but there has been a growing acknowledgment that mood problems do occur in the young. Furthermore, the accumulated data indicate that although depressive symptoms and Depressive Disorder in children clearly do show some developmental features, the overall conceptualizations of depression developed for adults also work for children and adolescents (Kashani, Holcomb, & Orvaschel, 1986; Ryan et al., 1987). Less is known about mania and Bipolar Disorders in children and adolescents (see below), but progress is being made in this area as well.

The "Mood Disorders" chapter of DSM-IV brings together most of the syndromes and disorders in this classification system where mood symptoms are the primary clinical problem. For children and adolescents, the principal additional categories are various forms of

Adjustment Disorder involving mood disturbance, and Bereavement (which is a V code and not a mental disorder). The next IDEA Note sets forth how these disorders and conditions relate to eligibility for services under IDEA.

Specific Mood Disturbance Patterns

Syndromes

DSM-IV defines several mood syndromes, which are then used in the criteria of several Mood Disorders. The mood syndromes identified

---

IDEA NOTE   Mood-Related Disorders/Conditions and IDEA

A DSM-IV diagnosis of a Mood Disorder (or other mental disorder or condition centering around mood) can be used to support qualifying a child for special services under the "seriously emotionally disturbed" category of IDEA. A "general pervasive mood of unhappiness or depression" that persists "over a period of time" and "adversely affects educational performance" is one of the identified conditions indicating "seriously emotionally disturbed" (U.S. Department of Health, Education and Welfare, 1977, p. 42478). Another identified condition is "an inability to build or maintain satisfactory relationships with peers and teachers," which is a common symptom of Mood Disorders in children and adolescents. Documentation of the functional impairment in academic or social adjustment caused by the mood disturbance will be important. The information on Axis IV (Psychosocial and Environmental Problems) and Axis V (Global Assessment of Functioning) may also be important in establishing eligibility for services under IDEA.

The IDEA description of severe emotional disturbance has been criticized on several grounds, including the requirement that the qualifying condition must have a negative impact on educational performance. It is certainly possible that a bright child could maintain adequate scholastic performance even under the burden of severe depression, for example, but typically depression will cause a decline in the quality of schoolwork. An unexplained deterioration in school performance is often an early overt symptom of MDD in children and adolescents. Clarizio and Payette's (1990) survey of school psychologists' practice with respect to childhood depression suggested a much greater reliance on the operational criteria of DSM-III-R than on P.L. 94-142. This probably continues to be the case with DSM-IV and IDEA.

---

are Major Depressive Episode, Manic Episode, Mixed Episode, and Hypomanic Episode.

MAJOR DEPRESSIVE EPISODE

The criteria for a Major Depressive Episode demarcate the boundaries of a serious depressive experience. Five of nine defining symptoms are required to be in evidence for a minimum of 2 weeks. These symptoms represent a change from the individual's previous level of functioning and cause either significant distress or functional impairment. One of the five or more symptoms used to document a Major Depressive Episode in a child or adolescent must be either (1) depressed or irritable mood (in adults, only depressed mood is considered) or (2) anhedonia (diminished pleasure or satisfaction in previously enjoyed activities). One of the remaining symptoms is also modified for children: Rather than the adult criterion of weight loss, the failure to show expected developmental weight gain can be considered a symptom of depression in children. There is discussion in the text of other developmental features of depression in youth. Somatic complaints, agitation and restlessness, and mood-congruent hallucinations may be more frequent in depression in prepubertal children. Adolescents may be more likely to show acting-out and conduct problems, substance misuse, and declining academic performance and achievement. Symptoms of mania preclude identification of a Major Depressive Episode, but symptoms of psychosis do not.

MANIC EPISODE

A Manic Episode is a period of "abnormally and persistently elevated, expansive, or irritable mood" (p. 328). Individuals who experience Manic Episodes tend to feel euphoric, self-confident, grandiose, and irritable; they seem to have endless energy, sleep little, and are busy almost constantly; poor judgement, excessive pursuit of pleasurable goals, and distractibility may seriously compromise their functional behavior. A Manic Episode is defined by the presence of the abnormal mood for at least 1 week, plus three or more of seven symptoms. Four symptoms are required if the mood is only irritable, as may be more typically the case in children and adolescents. Manic behavior in children may be more characterized by irritability and aggressive outbursts, and may be more chronic and continuous, than that seen in adults (Biederman, 1997). A Manic Episode is precluded by a Mixed Episode, but not by psychotic symptoms.

Manic symptoms that are elicited by antidepressant medication, electroconvulsive therapy, light therapy, or other drugs (e.g., corticosteroids) are not considered Manic Episodes and are not be used to document Bipolar I Disorder. If a child with MDD develops manic behavior in response to treatment with an antidepressant medication, the diagnosis of MDD remains, and a second diagnosis (Substance-Induced Mood Disorder, With Manic Features) is added. DSM-IV notes that such a response to somatic treatment may reflect a bipolar "diathesis" (p. 329), and that such an individual may have an increased likelihood of developing Bipolar I or Bipolar II Disorder in the future. Children and adolescents who show such a response to treatment should be monitored for possible future independent manic symptoms.

MIXED EPISODE

A Mixed Episode is a period of at least 1 week in which a person meets the criteria for both a Major Depressive Episode and a Manic Episode. The individual experiences labile and fluctuating moods and manifests symptoms of both depression and mania. Mixed Episodes may be more frequent in younger individuals. Mixed Episodes may develop out of a Major Depressive Episode or a Manic Episode, or may develop spontaneously. An episode of mixed symptoms that develops in response to a somatic treatment of depression is not considered a Mixed Episode and is not used to establish a diagnosis of Bipolar I Disorder (see "Manic Episode," above).

HYPOMANIC EPISODE

A Hypomanic Episode is a milder form of abnormally elevated mood. The criteria require only 4 days of distinctly different emotional experience characterized by a persistently expansive elevated, or irritable mood; plus three of seven additional symptoms (four if the mood disturbance is irritable). DSM-IV notes that Hypomanic Episodes in adolescents may be associated with truancy, delinquent behavior, school failure, or substance use. An episode of hypomanic symptoms in reaction to somatic treatment of depression is not considered a Hypomanic Episode and is not used to establish a diagnosis of Bipolar II Disorder (see "Manic Episode," above).

Mood Disorders

The initial concern about children and adolescents with Mood Disorders will often be precipitated by a change in the young persons' level of performance or adjustment. In particular, school psychologists mention motivational changes as a primary expression of depression in school settings (Clarizio & Payette, 1990). Deterioration in quality of academic performance, withdrawal from social and extracurricular activities, and/or the appearance of behavior problems in the absence of any history of acting out are examples of the negative changes in youth that both prompt caretaker concern and raise a question of possible mood disturbance. Although Mood Disorders in children may be less episodic than in adults, even so a recent change in a child's adjustment is an important cue. Even with more enduring presentations (e.g., Dysthymic Disorder) we are often rewarded for asking this question: "Has the child always been like this?"

ISSUES IN EVALUATION OF MOOD DISORDERS

Developmental Trends. Although there is evidence of significant correlations between various Mood Disorders, these patterns can be supported as distinct clinical phenomena in children (Keller, 1994; Simeon, 1989). An awareness of developmental trends is valuable, especially in school settings, where a child may be followed over years. Dysthymic Disorder often shows the earliest age of onset among the Mood Disorders and can be identified in some children as early as preschool (Kashani, Allan, Beck, Bledsoe, & Reid, 1997). Some cases of Dysthymic Disorder follow a continuous or intermittent course throughout an individual's life, whereas others evolve into other Mood Disorder patterns. The earlier the onset of the Dysthymic Disorder, the greater the comorbidity of other mental disorders. In approximately 70% of cases of early-onset Dysthymic Disorder, the young person will eventually develop MDD (Birmaher et al., 1996). MDD tends to be episodic; the Dysthymic Disorder may or may not be evident during periods of recovery from the MDD. Finally, between 20% and 40% of adolescents with a diagnosis of MDD will develop Bipolar I Disorder within 5 years (Birmaher et al., 1996).

Developmental trends are also evident in the emerging literature on Bipolar Disorders in children and adolescents. As just noted, a number of adolescents with an initial presentation of depression will eventually "switch" to a manic symptom picture. In adolescents, the manic presentation is often an adult-pattern onset—abrupt, discontinuous with previous adjustment, responsive to treatment, and fully resolved between episodes (Geller & Luby, 1997). The presentation in children may be more insidious and chronic, with rapid cycling a prominent feature (Geller & Luby, 1997); this has undoubtedly contributed to the limited recognition of and underdiagnosis of Bipolar Disorders in youth.

Comorbidity. Comorbidity is the rule rather than the exception for Mood Disorders as defined by DSM-IV, complicating the task for the examiner. Birmaher et al.'s (1996) recent review reported that among youth with MDD 40–70% have another psychiatric diagnosis, with 20–50% having two or more comorbid diagnoses. The most frequently reported comorbid disorders with MDD are Dysthymic Disorder, Anxiety Disorders, ADHD and other Disruptive Behavior Disorders, and Substance-Related Disorder. Especially for other internalizing disorders, it may be especially difficult to establish a clear case for asserting an independent diagnosis, as opposed to considering the other internalizing symptoms as associated symptoms of the MDD. The methodological difficulties associated with evaluating emotional problems versus conduct disturbances in children are another major stumbling block here, and often only repeated assessments involving multiple informants can clarify the clinical picture. The overall directive is relatively clear: Isolated symptoms of anxiety can be considered associated symptoms of MDD; an Anxiety Disorder, however, should be recognized if it is occurring and diagnosed if it meets full criteria.

A recent review of Bipolar Disorders in children and adolescents (Geller & Luby, 1997) noted similar high frequencies of comorbidity with other behavior problems. Among children seen for evaluation of Bipolar Disorders almost 90% have a history of ADHD; among adolescents the prevalence is 30% (Geller et al., 1995). Conduct Disorder has been diagnosed in approximately 22% of children and 18% of adolescents evaluated with a Bipolar Disorder (Geller et al., 1995). These results raise conceptual questions: Are ADHD and the Disruptive Behavior Disorders seen in youth prior to a diagnosis of a Bipolar Disorder the initial presentation of the mood disorder or separate comorbid conditions? The high reported comorbidities also present challenges for differential diagnosis. Anxiety Disorders are common in children (33%) and adolescents (12%) with Bipolar Disorders (Geller et al., 1995). Given the multiple and frequent associations between manic behavior and other difficulties, it is very important to consider other possible diagnoses when evaluating the youth who presents with evidence of a Bipolar Disorder.

Quantifying the subjective experience of mood through the use of mood rating scales or other self-report scales can be very helpful in monitoring the course of Mood Disorders. Agreement between child and parent reports are poor for Mood Disorders (Cantwell et al, 1997), and positive reports of symptoms from young people themselves should probably be weighted more heavily than negative reports of symptoms from caretakers.

Major Depressive Disorder

MDD (Major Depression in DSM-III and DSM-III-R) is diagnosed on the basis of a Major Depressive Episode's being fully manifested (five of nine criteria are required, as noted above) for 2 weeks or more in a child or adolescent. Comorbid diagnoses may be justified in severely depressed adolescents.

For a child, I recommend a differential consideration of possible MDD if the examiner is confronted with repeated somatic complaints without apparent explanation, a perception by others (teacher, parents, peers) that the child is unhappy or seems sad, or an unexplained deterioration in school performance or behavior. My index of sensitivity is markedly increased in cases where there is a family history of Mood Disorder. Anxiety is a frequently associated symptom of depression in children and adolescents (Tumuluru, Yaylayan, Weller, & Weller, 1996a). Any prior history of serious depression is a significant risk factor for subsequent clinical depressions. MDD is specified as Single Episode or Recurrent. Whereas the Single Episode type is a risk factor for future depression, the Recurrent type almost guarantees recurrence of Major Depressive Episodes over the life span and justifies appropriate planning.

A specifier available in DSM-IV for MDD is With Seasonal Pattern. More commonly referred to as "seasonal affective disorder," the occurrence of some severe depressions at particular times of the year (usually fall or winter) is now well accepted. Often associated with excessive sleeping, overeating, craving for carbohydrate-rich foods, and weight gain, seasonal affective disorder has gained increasing attention in investigations of recurrent depressions in adults but little systematic study in children (Giedd, Swedo, Lowe, & Rosenthal, 1998). Despite the limited empirical literature, there is good reason to conclude that seasonal affective disorder does occur in children and is often missed in evaluations. Giedd et al. (1998) present a case series of youngsters followed over 7 years with diagnoses of seasonal affective disorder. They suggest that a pattern of best school performance in the first and last quarters, with deterioration of academic achievement in the second and third quarters, may indicate the presence of this disorder. Their literature review suggests a 3% estimated prevalence of seasonal affective disorder in children; the majority of these cases are not diagnosed. Sensitivity to this diagnostic possibility could be a valuable service of the school psychologist.

DYSTHYMIC DISORDER

Dysthymic Disorder (Dysthymia or Depressive Neurosis in DSM-III and DSM-III-R) identifies a chronic depressive state of less severity than the more florid MDD. As with MDD, important developmental modifications for Dysthymic Disorder in children and adolescents have been made in both the defining mood criteria and the duration criteria. The negative mood, as in MDD, can be one of either depression or irritability (depressed mood is required in adults); in addition, the duration required for diagnosis is reduced from 2 years (for adults) to 1 year. During the period of negative mood, two out of a list of six additional symptoms are required. Kashani et al. (1997) discuss the relative usefulness of different sources of informants (child, parent, teacher) in gathering data on dysthymic symptoms in very young children. Especially in younger children, the presentation of Dysthymic Disorder may differ for the typical clinical picture. Kashani's group found psychomotor agitation, aggressive behavior, and somatic complaints (none of which are DSM-IV symptoms of Dysthymic Disorder) to be very common in a group of preschool children diagnosed with this disorder (75%, 100%, and 100%, respectively; Kasani et al., 1997, p. 1431). In contrast, decreased physical activity (which is given as an alternative Criterion B symptom for Dysthymic Disorders in Appendix B of DSM-IV) occurred in only 25% of this sample of preschool children.

During the 1-year duration of Dysthymic Disorder required in children and adolescents, it is specified that a young person must never have been free from symptoms for a period of 2 months or more. The development of a full-blown Major Depressive Episode at any time during the initial year of Dysthymic Disorder preempts the diagnosis of DD, and the youth is diagnosed with MDD instead. After the 1-year "qualifying period" for Dysthymic Disorder, a Major Depression superimposed on Dysthymic Disorder receives a second diagnosis (Dysthymic Disorder and MDD); in much of the psychological literature, this situation is referred to as "dual depression." Appearance of a Manic Episode, Mixed Episode, or Hypomanic Episode preempts the diagnosis of DD, and the diagnosis of either Bipolar I or Bipolar II Disorder is given instead; any history of Cyclothymic Disorder preempts the diagnosis of DD.

DEPRESSIVE DISORDER NOT OTHERWISE SPECIFIED

Depressive Disorder NOS is a residual category for clinical pictures of depression that do not meet the requirements for any of the identified patterns in DSM-IV. This diagnosis is not made concurrently with that of another specific Mood Disorder. The presence of atypical features or symptoms may be noted after a specific Mood Disorder, but these should not be classified as a separate additional diagnosis. Depressive Disorder NOS can be diagnosed in association with other general groups of Axis I diagnoses if the depressive symptoms are not common associated symptoms of that disorder. For instance, Depressive Disorder NOS may be diagnosed in association with OCD. Depressive Disorder NOS should not be diagnosed concurrently with Schizophrenia, however, because depressive symptoms are commonly associated features of this Psychotic Disorder.

BIPOLAR I DISORDER, BIPOLAR II DISORDER, CYCLOTHYMIC DISORDER, AND BIPOLAR DISORDER NOT OTHERWISE SPECIFIED

Manic Episodes are rare in children (<1% of cases; Biederman, 1997; Emslie, Kennard, & Kowatch, 1995) and not very common in adolescents However, they do occur, and they are probably often missed because of evaluators failure to consider them possibilities. Bipolar I Disorder involves a current episode or past history of at least one full-blown criteria Manic Episode; there may or may not be a history of Major Depressive Episodes. Bipolar II Disorder involves a current episode or past history of at least one Major Depressive and at least one Hypomanic Episode (mild manic syndrome). Cyclothymic Disorder in children and adolescents involves at least 1 year of "numerous periods of hypomanic symptoms" and "numerous periods of depressive symptoms" that never meet full criteria for a Manic Episode or a Major Depressive Episode. After the 1-year period has passed, a concurrent diagnosis of Cyclothymic Disorder and either MDD or Bipolar I Disorder can be made. Bipolar Disorder NOS covers a number of possible combinations of mood symptoms that do not meet the criteria for any specific Bipolar Disorder.

Differential Diagnosis. Emslie et al. (1995) and Geller and Luby (1997) discuss reasons why Bipolar Disorders are difficult to diagnose in childhood and adolescence, and give examples of behavior in children that reflect the DSM-IV criteria for these disorders. Earlier, Weinberg and Brumback (1976) presented alternative criteria for mania in children. A review of this material may be helpful in sensitizing an examiner to possible signs of manic behavior, but a formal diagnosis of Bipolar Disorder requires the documentation of symptoms that meet the DSM-IV criteria.

The differential diagnosis of Bipolar Disorders versus ADHD has become an issue with increased consideration of possible Bipolar Disorders in adolescents. Bipolar Disorders in adolescents are expected to be episodic and relatively uninfluenced by environmental settings and contingencies; ADHD, in contrast, tends to be a consistent problem, but does clearly vary in response to situation and feedback. The situation is complicated by the evidence that ADHD and Bipolar Disorders may be associated (Biederman, 1997). There have been cases reported that initially presented as ADHD and later appeared to develop into a Bipolar Disorder (Tumuluru, Yaylayan, Weller, & Weller, 1996b). Birmaher et al. (1996) feel that greater attention to the possibility of Bipolar II Disorder in adolescents is important, because the symptoms of this Mood Disorder can easily be mistaken for those of a Disruptive Behavior Disorder or a Personality Disorder, especially Borderline Personality Disorder. Geller and Luby (1997), in the review discussed previously, argue that Bipolar Disorders are underdiagnosed in children because of age-specific developmental features in presentation and course.

The differentiation of Bipolar Disorders from Schizophrenia in adolescents (and possibly children) can be problematic as well. Adolescent-onset mania may present more often with psychotic symptoms that are misdiagnosed as Schizophrenia (McGlashan, 1988). Werry (1996, p. 33) has suggested that the following features are more common in child and adolescent psychosis due to Bipolar Disorders (as opposed to Schizophrenia): (1) lack of developmental abnormalities, (2) acute (rapid) onset, and (3) a family history of Bipolar Disorders. Geller and Luby (1997) also stress a family history of mania as an important aid in differentiating Bipolar Disorders from Schizophrenia in adolescents.

Other possibilities to be considered in the differential diagnosis of Bipolar Disorders in teenagers are the Substance-Related Disorders. Both can lead to abrupt changes in usual behavior, emotional symptoms, and deteriorating adjustment and school performance. This challenge is further complicated by the possibility that Bipolar Disorders in youth may occur more characteristically with rapid cycling, and hence may be less distinct from the "highs" and "lows" produced by substance use. Moreover, there is a high comorbidity between actual bipolar Disorder and Substance-Related Disorders; in particular many adolescents with Bipolar I Disorder will begin or increase substance use along with the other behavior excesses of a Manic Episode. A very careful review of a young person's substance use history, with multiple informants if possible, is strongly advised in any evaluation for possible Bipolar Disorders in youth.

Geller and Luby (1997) recommend that young people being

evaluated for possible Bipolar Disorders also be evaluated for possible Communication Disorders. A young person may present with disorganized speech that suggests a thought disorder but actually reflects a primary language disturbance. The child's or adolescent's need to communicate and frantic attempts to do so may be interpreted as a flight of ideas or pressured speech. Youth with manic symptoms are highly distractible and can show looseness of associations, but do not have any fundamental language problem.

A final consideration for differential diagnosis of Bipolar Disorders involves a presentation of hypersexual behavior. Excessive goal-directed activity is a cardinal symptom of mania, and one common manifestation is an increase in sexual speech, sexual behavior, and sexual acting out. Uncharacteristic profanity, poorly concealed masturbation, ill-considered propositioning of potential sexual partners, romantic fantasies with delusional qualities, use of telephone sex services ("1-900" calls), and dangerous sexual behavior (unprotected sex, multiple partners, little or no discrimination in selection of sexual partners) may all be symptomatic of a Manic Episode in older children and adolescents. These behaviors may also reflect a history of sexual abuse, and a careful evaluation of this possibility is called for whenever the school psychologist is confronted with unusual sexual activity in a young person.

Heuristic for Suspecting Mania in Children and Adolescents. A positive family history of Bipolar Disorders is strongly associated with manic–depressive behavior (Isaac, 1991), and Bipolar Disorders should be included among the diagnostic considerations in any child or adolescent with such a family history. In addition, I recommend a consideration of Bipolar Disorders in children exhibiting disruptive behavior who are also reported to have exhibited the following characteristics:

1. Sustained, chronic irritable moods.
2. Labile, unstable moods.
3. Incidents of explosive aggression that are poorly organized and seem nonfunctional.
4. Poor response to usually effective treatments.
5. A history of ADHD diagnosis with fluctuating symptoms or responses to treatment.

OTHER MOOD DISORDERS

Mood Disorder in children and adolescents can develop as a consequence of substance use (Substance-Induced Mood Disorder) or a general medical condition (Mood Disorder Due to a General Medical Condition). That is, symptoms of depression, mania, or both may develop during drug or medication intoxication or withdrawal, as well as in response to illness, injury, or some other physiological influence. Finally, Mood Disorder NOS can be diagnosed for a clinical picture that (1) meets the general criteria for a mental disorder; (2) does not meet the criteria for any specific Depressive or Bipolar Disorder; and (3) involves both manic and depressive symptoms, but neither appears to predominate.

Other Mood-Related Disorders/Conditions

ADJUSTMENT DISORDERS INVOLVING MOOD DISTURBANCE

As noted previously, an Adjustment Disorder is a Mental Disorder; that is, it must fall within the general parameters of a Mental Disorder as defined by DSM-IV (clinically significant distress, impairment of adaptive behavior, or specific outcome risks). Adjustment Disorders in general are defined by the development of clinically significant symptoms in response to an identified psychosocial stress or stressors. Adjustment Disorders are excluded if the symptoms meet the criteria for an alternative, specific Axis I disorder, even if this disorder is precipitated by a known stressor. Adjustment Disorders in DSM-IV are classifications of exclusion; only if no other Axis I pattern accounts for the symptoms seen is an Adjustment Disorder diagnosis allowed. Adjustment Disorders can be diagnosed concurrently with other Axis I or II diagnoses, but only when novel problems have developed, that are not associated with the Axis I or II mental disorders and that are judged to be elicited by a clear precipitating event.

Adjustment Disorder is subtyped by the predominant symptoms experienced. Three of the five specific subtypes are relevant to this section: Adjustment Disorder With Depressed Mood, Adjustment Disorder With Mixed Anxiety and Depressed Mood, and Adjustment Disorder With Mixed Disturbance of Emotions <depression, anxiety> and Conduct. There is also an Unspecified subtype to cover other behavioral reactions. The diagnosis of Adjustment Disorder is usually not made if the symptom picture of depression occurs in response to a death; rather, the V code of Bereavement is given.

BEREAVEMENT

Bereavement is a V code (i.e., it is not a mental disorder as defined in DSM-IV, but is included in the chapter "Other Conditions That May

Be a Focus of Clinical Attention"). Bereavement is given somewhat more detailed treatment than most of the other V codes, in an effort to help differentiate between normal and psychopathological grief reactions. This discussion emphasizes symptoms that are not typically seen in normal grief. In general, the differential diagnosis of MDD versus Bereavement requires consideration of the symptoms presented; the survivor's expressed distress and personal interpretation of the symptoms experienced; the functional status of the survivor with respect to his or her major obligations (school, family responsibilities, social relationships); the survivor's cultural and family background; the survivor's relationship with the deceased; and the duration and course of the survivor's reaction to the death.

Horowitz et al. (1997) have proposed a new category, "complicated grief disorder," which would cover prolonged and turbulent grief reactions. This proposed category would be a Mental Disorder, in contrast to Bereavement. Although there seems to be some merit to their proposal for a diagnostic category of pathological grief, such a diagnosis was not included in DSM-IV. The cases they discuss would probably be classified as Depressive Disorder NOS or possibly Anxiety Disorder NOS in DSM-IV.

OTHER INTERNALIZING PROBLEMS

Several remaining groups of problems fall within the empirical cluster usually identified as "internalizing" or "overcontrolled" patterns. These include concerns and problems with a physical focus but without apparent medical basis, complaints that are primarily motivated by psychological needs, and disturbances in the integrity of the sense of self or other executive functions. In general, these disturbances in children and adolescents have received less empirical study than the other internalizing disorders, and less is known with confidence about them. To some extent, this reflects their lower base rate among clinical (and presumably the general) child and adolescent populations; however, it also reflects a greater lack of basic consensus among investigators and practitioners about the nature and even the reality of these phenomena in youth.

Somatoform Disorders

Somatoform Disorders present with physical symptoms or concerns that are not completely explained by general medical conditions. In contrast to Factitious Disorders and Malingering (see below), there is no indication that clients are deliberately faking, lying or misrepresenting their experience. They appear to be sincerely experiencing the difficulties they are reporting to their physicians, but a full understanding of their problems cannot be achieved on the basis of the demonstrable physical findings. Somatoform Disorders also differ from Psychological Factors Affecting Medical Condition (see below), in which there is a medical condition that can be diagnosed.

It is difficult to state with any confidence how common these phenomena may be, especially in children and adolescents. A general recommendation would be for evaluators to be very conservative with respect to Somatoform Disorder diagnoses. The consequences of missing a general medical condition may be much more serious than the consequences of delaying acceptance of a Somatoform Disorder diagnosis. At a minimum, a Somatoform Disorder diagnosis should be a positive diagnosis; that is, it should be "ruled in" by the available data. Such a diagnosis should not be made solely on the basis of there being no readily apparent biological basis for the problems; there must also be positive evidence that psychological factors do have a significant role in the difficulties. Mrazek (1994) has reviewed difficulties in basing diagnoses on the absence of physical explanations for symptoms.

Examiners would also do well to remember that there is nothing about manifesting a Somatoform Disorder that ensures good physical health thereafter. When a child or adolescent has a well-documented Somatization Disorder, it is necessary to monitor his or her health very carefully, because caretakers are likely to assume that any new ache, pain, or limitation reported is another expression of the mental disorder. A distressingly high percentage of children diagnosed with Conversion Disorder, for example, have been found to have had a physical disorder that could account for their symptoms (Lehmkuhl, Blanz, Lehmkuhl, & Braum-Scharm, 1989). This is consistent with the adult literature, which reveals many patients diagnosed with Conversion Disorders to be eventually diagnosed with neurological disorders (Katon, 1993).

A related concern in using Somatoform Disorder diagnoses with adolescents and especially with children is the absence of developmentally appropriate diagnostic criteria and of any adequate research base for empirical classification. Fritz, Fritsch, and Hagino (1997) provide a nice review of recent work in this area, but point out that progress is still hampered by diagnostic criteria that were developed for adults and are often not useful for children and adolescents. This is clearly an area in great need of further study and development.

The next IDEA Note sets forth how Somatization Disorders relate to eligibility for services under IDEA.

Somatization Disorder

Somatization Disorder has been referred to in the past as "hysteria," "hysterical neurosis," or "Briquet's syndrome." The client presents multiple somatic complaints and symptoms that cannot be demonstrated to have a physiological basis. These complaints begin before the age of 30, occur over several years, and result in the seeking of medical treatment or in functional impairment; they must include four pain symptoms, two gastrointestinal symptoms, one sexual symptom, and one "pseudoneurological" symptom. Despite past theoretical assumptions, a covariation between Somatization Disorder and Histrionic Personality Disorder has not been demonstrated.

Somatization Disorder is usually diagnosed in adults, but the behaviors may have begun in adolescence or childhood. Fritz et al. (1997) suggest that the infrequency with which Somatization Disor-

---

IDEA NOTE   Somatoform Disorders and IDEA

A diagnosis of a Somatoform Disorder can form the basis for qualifying a child for special services under the "seriously emotionally disturbed" category of IDEA. One of the identified conditions indicating "seriously emotionally disturbed" is a "tendency to develop physical symptoms or fears associated with personal or school problems" that persists "over a period of time" and "adversely affects educational performance" (U.S. Department of Health, Education and Welfare, 1977, p. 42478). Severe somatoform symptoms fall within this condition. Another identified condition is "an inability to build or maintain satisfactory relationships with peers and teachers," which can be a consequence of Somatoform Disorders in children and adolescents. Documentation of the functional impairment caused by the Somatoform Disorder on academic or social adjustment will be important.

The information on Axis IV (Psychosocial and Environmental Problems) and Axis V (Global Assessment of Functioning) may also be important in establishing eligibility for services under IDEA. As previously discussed for anxiety and mood problems (see the IDEA Notes on pp. 63 and 78), it is necessary under IDEA to document the effect of an emotional disturbance on educational performance.

---

der is diagnosed in youth is the result of developmentally inappropriate criteria rather than the absence of the phenomenon. The literature on childhood depression suggests that young children often express emotional distress in terms of physical complaints. Nonspecific
abdominal pain and headaches are relatively frequent somatic symptoms in youth (Fritz et al., 1997). It is hoped that continued investigation will contribute more developmentally useful formations of somatization behavior in young people.

Undifferentiated Somatoform Disorder

Undifferentiated Somatization Disorder is a residual category to cover
cases having the general features of Somatization Disorder but not
meeting one or more of the specific criteria—in other words, sub-
threshold, unexplained physical complaints. Given the unsuitability
of some of the Somatization Disorder criteria for prepubertal children, this diagnostic category would potentially have some application to juvenile cases, but an available clinical or empirical literature
has yet to be developed. The category has recently received a new
ICD-9-CM code (see the following Coding Note).

Conversion Disorder

Conversion Disorder is characterized by the appearance of a problem with motor control or sensory functioning that would usually sug-

---

**CODING NOTE   Coding Changes for Undifferentiated
Somatoform Disorder and Somatoform Disorder NOS**

As mentioned earlier in this book (see the Coding Note on p. 49), the
ICD-9-CM is annually reviewed and updated by a federal committee.
Following the submission and review process described in that Coding Note, the final coding changes are published as an Interim Final
Notice in the May–June issue of the *Federal Register*. Two recent publications by the American Psychiatric Association (1996a, 1996b) present
23 updated codes affecting DSM-IV diagnostic categories and 7 updated codes from DSM-IV Appendix G. Two of the categories affected
are Undifferentiated Somatoform Disorder and Somatoform Disorder NOS. Previously both were coded as 300.81 in ICD-9-CM; both are
now coded as 300.82.

---

gest a neurological or other medical problem but is without demon-strable biological foundation. The symptom pattern is usually focused and relatively stable, in contrast to the many and fluctuating symptoms of Somatization Disorder and Undifferentiated Somatoform Disorder. Although case studies of Conversion Disorder have been the basis for much theoretical discussion, empirical studies are infrequent. Siegel and Barthel (1986) reported on the frequency of several characteris-tics of Conversion Disorder in a pediatric sample. They found evi-dence of an identifiable psychosocial stress in 89% of these cases, a model for conversion symptoms in 56%, and family dysfunction in 56%; there was evidence of secondary gain in 41% of these cases.

Classic Conversion Disorder, involving paralysis or loss of sen-sory functions (e.g., "hysterical paralysis" of the legs or "hysterical blindness"), seems relatively rare today in adults but continues to be seen occasionally in children. Conversion Disorder involving neuro-logical phenomena ("pseudoseizures") may be more common. DSM-IV suggests that conversion symptoms in children under the age of 10 usually involve gait problems or seizures. Fritz et al. (1997) report that pseudoseizures, partial paralysis, paresthesias, and gait distur-bances are the conversion symptoms most frequently reported in chil-dren. The diagnostic dilemma in child neurological cases may be great, due to the reported occurrence both of seizures with a clear neuro-logical basis and of pseudoseizures in the same children. Both care-ful evaluation and skillful intervention are required to manage and treat these children effectively. Wynick, Hobson, and Jones (1997) report that cases of psychogenic disorders of vision, or "visual conver-sion reactions," are often seen by ophthalmologists rather than men-tal health professionals; such cases tend to be related to environmen-tal stress, and respond well to suggestion or reassurance.

In my practice, Conversion Disorder in children and adolescents has usually been associated with significant family conflict and with inconsistency both in expectations for the youth and in consequences for behavior. There is often a precipitating stressor for the original manifestation of the problem, but this cannot always be identified with certainty. The waxing and waning of symptoms are usually asso-ciated with increased and decreased psychological stress within the young persons' family, school, and/or community experience. Asso-ciations with other somatoform symptoms and occasionally other Somatoform Disorders occur. Associations with dependent and op-positional personality traits can sometimes be seen. Comorbid or possible future diagnoses of MDD, Dysthymic Disorder, ODD or other Disruptive Behavior Disorders should be considered and ruled in or out. DSM-IV suggests that there may be associations with Histrionic,

Antisocial, and Dependent Personality Disorders; however, even if this is the case, these diagnoses usually cannot be made with confidence in a child or adolescent (Antisocial Personality Disorder cannot be diagnosed prior to age 18).

Both high suggestibility and secondary gain (positive or negative reinforcement, usually unintentional, of sick role behavior) are commonly found in children and adolescents with Conversion Disorder, but these characteristics have a very high base rate in the general population and in clinical populations. I do not believe that suggestibility or evidence of secondary gain can be used with any confidence to rule in Conversion Disorder. Similarly, an apparent lack of concern over symptoms (*la belle indifférence*) can be an associated feature of Conversion Disorder, but it too lacks adequate positive or negative predictive value to be accorded significant diagnostic weight. Siegel and Barthel (1986) found evidence of secondary gain in 41% of their cases and *la belle indifférence* in 30%.

Conversion Disorder is subclassified in terms of type of symptom or deficit: With Motor Symptom or Deficit, With Sensory Symptom or Deficit, With Seizures or Convulsions, or With Mixed Presentation.

Pain Disorder

Pain Disorder is diagnosed on Axis I in cases where psychological factors are believed to play some important role in the pain problems of a child or adolescent. There may also be physiological factors producing pain (a general medical condition), but severity, exacerbation, and/or maintenance of the pain is also significantly influenced by psychological variables. If there is little or no involvement of psychological factors, the diagnosis is Pain Disorder Associated With a General Medical Condition. This is *not* a mental disorder; it is coded on Axis III according to the location of the pain or the associated medical problem. Pain Disorder Associated With Psychological Factors and Pain Disorder Associated With Both Psychological Factors and a General Medical Condition are classified as Mental Disorders and are coded on Axis I. Pain Disorder can occur at all ages and is usually worked up within a medical setting. The conceptual and methodological issues and difficulties involved in dealing with pain in children and adolescents have received some attention in the literature (e.g., McGrath, 1995). Effective assessment and evaluation usually require cooperation among multiple specialists.

Hypochondriasis

Hypochondriasis is manifested in fears of and preoccupations with being ill. Hypochondriasis is almost always diagnosed in adults, but these adults often report histories of excessive interest in and concern over bodily states and symptoms stretching back into childhood. In my experience, children and adolescents who demonstrate frequent concerns about health in the absence of a history of critical health problems often have a family pattern of high sensitivity to possible illness and symptoms of illness. There may be a family history of a critical, debilitating, or fatal illness in a sibling or a child from a previous generation. A critical intervention goal is to help the young person and family avoid extinguishing appropriate adult concern to reports of potentially important physical symptoms.

Body Dysmorphic Disorder

Body Dysmorphic Disorder, or "dysmorphophobia" as it has traditionally been called in the literature," reflects a preoccupation with a perceived defect in bodily appearance. The concern is intense enough to cause significant personal distress or functional impairment (i.e., it meets criteria for a Mental Disorder). The onset of Body Dysmorphic Disorder is probably during adolescence, but most known cases involve adults. Careful review of how much time is spent in a day ruminating about or inspecting the offending body part(s), evaluation of the presence and intensity of anxiety symptoms, and especially assessment of avoidance behavior or social withdrawal because of the perceived ''deformity" are useful in establishing a clinical diagnosis.

Somatoform Disorder Not Otherwise Specified

Somatoform Disorder NOS is a residual diagnostic category for cases of Somatoform Disorder that do not fully meet the criteria for identified patterns. For example, "pseudocyesis" (a mistaken belief that one is pregnant, associated with some of the usual objective signs of pregnancy) is occasionally seen in adolescent females; such cases are diagnosed as Somatoform Disorder NOS. Somatoform Disorder NOS has recently received a new ICD-9-CM code (see the previous Coding Note on p. 92).

Other Mental Disorders/Conditions
Involving Presentation of Physical Symptoms

Psychological Factors Affecting Medical Condition

Psychological Factors Affecting Medical Condition is a V code (not a mental disorder) used to identify cases in which there are extant medical or physical problems in an individual's life, and there is also

evidence that psychological factors play a significant role in the exacerbation or maintenance of these medical difficulties. The role of
good clinical judgment is especially important with this category. Psychological factors probably play a role in most disease and recovery
courses, but this category is intended to note those instances where
the role is of marked importance in understanding cases and manag-
ing them effectively. Close cooperation and frequent communication
between the medical professionals involved and the school psychologist constitute the best basis for both identifying and responding help-
fully to these cases.

Noncompliance with Treatment

Noncompliance with Treatment is a V code (again, not a Mental Disorder) applicable to situations in which clinical attention needs to be
focused on the client's failure to cooperate with treatment. This noncompliance can be associated with normal child or adolescent development, with other situations that are best conceptualized in terms
of V codes (e.g., Parent–Child Relational Problem), or with a specific
mental disorder (e.g., Oppositional Defiant Disorder or Personality
Disorder NOS [passive–aggressive personality disorder]). Regardless
of the context, the matter is serious enough to warrant clinical attention and hence formal identification. The potential effects can range
from minor annoyances to life-threatening medical consequences
(e.g., a diabetic boy refuses to control his alcohol intake; a girl with
previously well-controlled phenylketonuria (PKU) will not adhere to
the dietary restrictions that set her apart from her peer group).

Factitious Disorder and Factitious Disorder Not Otherwise Specified

Factitious Disorder reflects the deliberate feigning of symptoms of a
Mental Disorder or General Medical Condition, with the only apparent motivation being that of assuming the role of patient. There is an
absence of clear external reinforcement (payoff) for the sick role.
The few times I have seen this behavior in adolescents, it was always
associated with other Mental Disorders on Axis I, Axis II, or both.
Factitious Disorder differs from Somatoform Disorders, where there
are also apparent physical symptoms without a biological basis, but
where the problems and complaints are not being intentionally and
knowingly concocted. Individuals with Factitious Disorder (like those
exhibiting Malingering) are aware of "putting on."

Factitious Disorder NOS includes cases that resemble Factitious
Disorder in some respects but do not meet the full criteria. These

include cases where the deception involves one person's claiming and/ or producing symptoms in another (usually a parent provoking unnecessary medical attention for a child)—"factitious disorder by proxy."

Malingering

Malingering is the V code used to classify intentional "faking" of symptoms or a disorder in order to achieve some desired end. It is the presence of an identifiable payoff or external incentive that differentiates Malingering from Factitious Disorder; it is the conscious, intentional aspect that differentiates Malingering from Conversion Disorder. A trivial manifestation in children and adolescents is feigning illness to avoid school for a day. Much more serious is feigning ADHD in order to obtain a prescription for a stimulant medication to be misused or resold.

Adjustment Disorder, Unspecified

Occasionally the psychologist will see physical complaints that have developed in response to psychosocial stress and appear to meet the general criteria of a Mental Disorder. These can be diagnosed as Adjustment Disorder, Unspecified.

Dissociative Disorders

Dissociative Disorders all reflect a "disruption in the usually integrated functions of consciousness, memory, identity, or perception of the environment" (p. 477). Although dissociative symptoms are very common in both normal development and many mental disorders, I would advise caution in making a Dissociative Disorder diagnosis in children or adolescents, especially as a primary diagnosis. Great controversy surrounds this topic, and unfortunately "more heat than light" is currently being offered in much of the available literature on both sides of the controversy. The development of instruments such as the Child Dissociative Checklist, a parent report dissociative checklist (Putnam et al., 1993), and the Adolescent Dissociative Experiences Scale, an adolescent self-report measure (Armstrong et al., 1997), may help guide clinical evaluation in this area—as similar checklists have helped move the assessment of attention deficits onto a more objective and empirically based foundation. The next IDEA Note sets forth how Dissociative Disorders relate to eligibility for services under IDEA.

IDEA NOTE   Dissociative Disorders and IDEA

Although dissociative experiences appear to be relatively common and unremarkable in children, severe and enduring dissociative phenomena that cause marked distress or impair social or academic adjustment (i.e., Dissociative Disorders) are rare among children and adolescents, in my experience. If a severe Dissociative Disorder is diagnosed in a young person, it can probably serve as the basis for eligibility for services under IDEA through several of the conditions identifying "severely emotionally disturbed." If dissociative symptoms interfere with learning, they can meet the criterion of "an inability to learn which cannot be explained by intellectual, sensory, or health factors." If dissociative symptoms interfere with social relationships, they can thus cause "an inability to build or maintain satisfactory relationships with peers and teachers." Finally, if dissociative symptoms lead to socially deviant actions or unusual emotional responses, they therefore result in "inappropriate types of behavior or feelings under normal circumstances" (U.S. Department of Health, Education and Welfare, 1977, p. 42478). As previously discussed for anxiety and mood problems (see the two IDEA Notes on pp. 63 and 78), it is necessary under IDEA to document the effect of an emotional disturbance on educational performance.

Dissociative Amnesia

Dissociative Amnesia (Psychogenic Amnesia in DSM-III and DSM-III-R) refers to loss of important personal information that is too excessive for normal forgetting and not accounted for by another Dissociative Disorder, PTSD, Acute Stress Disorder, Somatization Disorder, or an Amnestic Disorder. Symptoms of dissociative amnesia occur in children and adolescents, often as part of the clinical picture of a trauma reaction. DSM-IV notes that differential diagnosis of Dissociative Amnesia in children is complicated by several developmental features, and multiple sources of data are often necessary (p. 479).

Dissociative Fugue

Dissociative Fugue (Psychogenic Fugue in DSM-III and DSM-III-R) consists of a person's leaving his or her usual setting, traveling some distance, and setting up a new life, accompanied with confusion about or amnesia for his or her previous identity and often assumption of a new identity. The problem is rare in general, and even more so in adolescents; onset is usually associated with traumatic events or overwhelming stress. Careful evaluation is needed to rule out Malingering, Psychotic Disorders, Manic Episodes, and neurological disorders with complex partial (temporal lobe or psychomotor) seizures.

Dissociative Identity Disorder

Dissociative Identity Disorder (DID; Multiple Personality Disorder in DSM-III-R, Multiple Personality in DSM-III) is still often referred to by the acronym MPD for Multiple Personality Disorder, the historical label for the phenomenon. A related concept is "false-memory syndrome," an expression used by those who challenge the validity of the frequent use of DID as an explanation for difficult-to-understand clinical cases. The DSM-IV label change is very welcome to those of us who were uncomfortable with the idea of one body having more than one personality, but can accept the idea of one body having more than one identity. There are more than semantic niceties at stake here; issues of criminal responsibility, the validity of "recovered memories," the choice of acceptable therapeutic goals, and other critical concerns are at stake. This diagnostic category marks one set of limits about what we understand regarding the development and vicissitudes of a human's sense of self, identity, and personality. It is a small part of the answer to questions about when and under what circumstances a person should feel and be held accountable for the actions his or her body takes.

I would usually recommend that diagnoses of DID in children or adolescents only be made after consultation with colleagues. All major discussions in the literature I have seen acknowledge the frequent association of DID with Mood Disorders, Anxiety Disorders, Personality Disorders, Eating Disorders, Substance-Related Disorders, Sexual and Gender Identity Disorders, and occasionally Psychotic Disorders. In particular, comorbid diagnoses with PTSD, Substance-Related Disorders, MDD, and Borderline Personality Disorder occur with some regularity. Although I am convinced that dissociative phenomena are real, the clinical utility of DID as a diagnostic category (rather than a therapeutic metaphor—an "as if you were") is not well established, in my view. Nevertheless, it is available as a diagnosis in DSM-IV, and the phenomenon is reported in children and adolescents. Kluft (1984) provided some data on children who received a DSM-III diagnosis of Multiple Personality.

Child battering, sexual exploitation and abuse, and/or neglect of basic developmental needs are common problems of pathological parenting reported to be associated with DID. DSM-IV includes the following three problems in the "Other Conditions That May Be a Focus of Clinical Attention" chapter: Physical Abuse of Child, Sexual Abuse of Child, or Neglect of Child. I discuss these conditions further in Chapter 6 of this book.

Identity Problem

Another V code, Identity Problem, should be mentioned briefly in this context. Identify Problem is used to classify problems with identity issues such as goals, career direction, sexual orientation, or religious beliefs. Several such concerns are common developmental issues of adolescence and early adulthood, and such concerns are not usually viewed as indicative of a mental disorder unless the distress or functional impairment is significant. Identity Problem is seldom in question when symptoms of DID are at issue, but it is mentioned here because the similarity of title can be confusing.

Depersonalization Disorder

As its names indicates, Depersonalization Disorder involves episodes of depersonalization—feelings of detachment or unreality regarding one's self. Occasional feelings of depersonalization are common both in normal adolescents and in adolescents with a wide variety of mental disorders. A diagnosis of Depersonalization Disorder is only made if the symptoms are frequent and intense enough to cause significant distress and/or impairment (i.e., constitute a mental disorder), *and* if they occur independently of another mental disorder.

Dissociative Disorder Not Otherwise Specified

Dissociative Disorder NOS is used to classify a variety of unusual case presentations, dissociative trance disorders (culture bound phenomena), and atypical cases similar to DID. The following Professional Note describes a condition called "dissociative hallucinosis" that appears to fall into this category.

PROFESSIONAL NOTE   Dissociative Hallucinosis

Nurcombe et al. (1996) discuss a condition they refer to as "dissociative hallucinosis," which appears to be a state with characteristics of Dissociative Disorders, Psychotic Disorders, and PTSD. Nurcombe and colleagues believe that there is a consistent phenomenon underlying a number of historical terms in psychopathology: "hysterical psychosis, hysterical hallucinations, hysterical twilight state, hysterical delirium, hysterical trance, hysterical pseudopsychosis, hysterical pseudoschizophrenia, hysterical pseudodementia, hypnoid state, somnambulistic crisis, psychological automatism, transient psychotic episode, episodic dyscontrol, and dissociative psychosis" (1996, p. 109). They identify defining features (1996, p. 110):

1. Acute onset, brief duration, and a recurrent course, but no personality deterioration.
2. Trance-like episodes of altered consciousness.
3. Hyperarousal and negative emotions (fear, anger).
4. Impulsive aggression, destructiveness, suicidal behavior, or self-injurious behavior.
5. Auditory and/or visual hallucinations, intrusive mental images, and nightmares.
6. Disorganized thinking.

The reliability and diagnostic/therapeutic validity of such a category remain to be convincingly demonstrated. The most appropriate DSM-IV diagnosis would probably be Dissociative Disorder NOS. I would recommend evaluating carefully to rule out (or in) Borderline Personality Disorder, which can show similar symptoms: transient psychotic episodes, including vivid hallucinations; acute confusion and disorientation; intense negative affect; self-injurious, aggressive, and destructive actions; and dissociative phenomena.

CHAPTER 6

Substance-Related Problems, Other "Addictive" Behaviors, and Harmful Environmental Effects

♦

SUBSTANCE-RELATED PROBLEMS

Overview

The Substance-Related Disorders in DSM-IV include disorders result-ing not only from deliberate use of a drug of abuse, but also from side effects of medication and unintentional exposure to a toxic. The term "substance" in DSM-IV can refer to a drug (including alcohol), a medication, or toxin. The "Substance-Related Disorders" chapter defines two broad groups: Substance Use Disorders and Substance-Induced Disorders. After syndromes within each of these two are de-fined, the chapter is then organized around 11 classes of substances plus two residual classes, Polysubstance and Other (or Unknown) Substance (see the following Coding Note). Some specific Substance-Induced Disorders are included in the chapters with phenomeno-logically related mental disorders (e.g., Substance-Induced Psychotic Disorder is found in the "Schizophrenia and Other Psychotic Disor-ders" chapter, Substance-Induced Anxiety Disorder is discussed in the "Anxiety Disorders" chapter, etc.). Although I focus primarily on the Substance-Related Disorders in this section, I also briefly mention several types of medication-induced problems that DSM-IV includes in the "Other Conditions That May Be a Focus of Clinical Attention" chapter.

CODING NOTE   Classes of Substances Discussed in DSM-IV

Alcohol	Nicotine
Amphetamines	Opioids
(or amphetamine-like substance)	Phencyclidine (or
Caffeine	phencyclidine-like substance)
Cannabis	Sedatives, hypnotics, or
Cocaine	anxiolytics
Hallucinogens	Polysubstance
Inhalants	Other (or unknown) substance

"Polysubstance" refers to at least three different groups of substances (other than caffeine and nicotine). Examples of other (or unknown) substances include anabolic steroids, nitrite inhalants ("poppers"), nitrous oxide ("laughing gas"), various over-the-counter and prescription medications not covered in other categories, and most environmental toxins.

Substance-Related Disorders

Substance Use Disorders

Substance Use Disorders are conceptualized in terms of two broad syndromes: Substance Abuse and Substance Dependence. Simply described, both represent problematic patterns of substance use; Substance Dependence is a more serious or dysfunctional pattern than Substance Abuse. The fact that there is no agreed upon definition of "alcoholism" testifies to the difficulty of establishing clear, categorical boundaries around psychopathological involvement with chemicals. The two-category system of DSM-IV can be faulted from several points of view, but overall it appears as workable (and as problematic) as any other classification that has been proposed. The next IDEA Note sets forth how Substance Use Disorders relate to eligibility for services under IDEA.

SUBSTANCE DEPENDENCE

Substance Dependence is a history of maladaptive substance use involving at least three of seven symptoms over the same 12-month period. Two of the seven symptoms (tolerance and withdrawal) evoke the specifier With Physiological Dependence, while their absence

---

IDEA NOTE   Substance Use Disorders and IDEA

Substance Use Disorders are not included in the list of disability conditions identified as elibible for services under IDEA. However, it appears that Substance Use Disorder can serve as the basis for a qualification through the "other health impaired" category, especially with documentation of how the Substance Use Disorder adversely affects educational adjustment and performance.

---

among the symptoms used to document Substance Dependence is specified as Without Physiological Dependence. As noted above, 11 classes of substances are given, as well as Polysubstance Dependence and Other (or Unknown) Substance Dependence.

Six course specifiers provide further details regarding the youth's current status if there is a history of Substance Dependence. Two identify treatments that may currently be bringing the Substance Dependence under control: On Agonist Therapy and In a Controlled Environment. Four other specifiers describe remissions: Early Full Remission (no criteria have been met for either Substance Dependence or Substance Abuse for at least 1 month but less than 12 months), Early Partial Remission (for at least 1 month but less than 12 months, one or more criteria for Abuse or Dependence have been met, but not the full criteria for either), Sustained Full Remission (no criteria for Dependence or Abuse have been met for more than 12 months), and Sustained Partial Remission (one or more Abuse or Dependence criteria, but full criteria for neither, have been met for more than 12 months). The figures on page 180 of the manual diagram the specifiers. Remission specifiers can only be used after a 1-month period in which the young person no longer meets full criteria for Substance Dependence or Substance Abuse. In addition, if the On Agonist Therapy or In a Controlled Setting specifier applies, the remission specifiers cannot be used until the treatment has been discontinued for at least 1 month.

SUBSTANCE ABUSE

Substance Abuse is manifested by one (or more) of four symptoms indicating that substance use is impairing the individual's adjustment. Substance Abuse has been a more problematic diagnosis than Substance Dependence in previous editions of DSM, and appears to continue to be so in DSM-IV (Hasin, McCloud, Qun, & Endicott, 1996). This may in part derive naturally from the intermediate place Substance Abuse takes between the more extreme psychopathology of Substance Dependence and nonpathological levels of substance use. The boundaries of substance use and Substance Abuse are sometimes not clear-cut, especially with adolescents (Newcomb & Bentler, 1989). Substance Abuse is only appropriate as a diagnosis if the youth has never met criteria for Substance Dependence of the class of substance under consideration. For example, once a teenager has been diagnosed with Alcohol Dependence, a single symptom from the Substance Abuse criterion set does not lead to a diagnosis of Alcohol Abuse, even after a period of Sustained Full Remission; instead, it is treated as a relapse of the Alcohol Dependence. The same adolescent can receive a diagnosis of Cannabis Abuse if he or she has never before met criteria for Cannabis Dependence. The diagnosis of Substance Abuse can be made with respect to 9 of the 11 classes of substances identified for Substance Dependence; a diagnosis of Substance Abuse is not made for the classes of caffeine and nicotine. There is also a category of Other (or Unknown) Substance Abuse. Course specifiers are not identified for Substance Abuse as "early" versus "sustained." The distinction between "partial remission" and "full remission" is not applicable, since a single symptom supports the diagnosis of Substance Abuse.

COMORBIDITY

A number of other mental disorders appear to increase the risk of Substance Abuse or Dependence, and Substance Abuse and Dependence seem to precipitate other mental disorders. Mood Disorders, Anxiety Disorders, and Disruptive Behavior Disorders show some linkage to problematic involvement with alcohol and other drugs. In turn, the abuse of alcohol or several other classes of drugs is a risk factor for depression, suicide attempts, and acting out. Alcohol use without permission has been linked in youth to increased risk for later abuse of other drugs and for other psychiatric diagnoses (Federman, Costello, Angold, Farmer, & Erkanli, 1997; Greenbaum, Foster-Johnson, & Petrila, 1996). As previously discussed in Chapter 4, early conduct problems or diagnosed Conduct Disorder is a risk factor for Substance Use Disorders in adolescence (Lynskey & Fergusson, 1995). Comorbidity with other mental disorders appears to have little impact on the course of Substance Use Disorders in adolescence, whereas comorbidity with Substance Use Disorders tends to have a significant and negative prognostic impact on other mental disorders in youth (Lewinsohn, Rohde, & Seeley, 1995).

Alcohol and most illicit drugs affect mood, impulse control, or both, so it should not be surprising to find high comorbidities reported between Substance Use Disorders and many other psychiatric conditions. Child and adolescents with Substance Use Disorders or subclinical problematic use of alcohol or illicit drugs should be carefully screened for other mental health problems. Beginning in adolescence, if not before, there are positive covariations between Alcohol/Drug Abuse/Dependence, Disruptive Behavior Disorders (CD, ODD, ADHD), and Learning Disorders. Indeed, the Substance Use Disorders join the childhood triad of conduct problems, hyperactivity, and learning problems, with a negative impact on at least short-term prognosis. The association between Substance Use Disorders and Mood Disorders is almost as strong; in particular, problems with Depressive Disorders may precede, occur concurrently with, and follow substance use problems in youth. Of particular concern is the association between alcohol/drug use and suicide in adolescents (Berman & Schwartz, 1990). Use of alcohol (or any other substance that impairs judgment and impulse control) is a risk factor for both suicide attempts and death (Spirito, Brown, Overholser, & Fritz, 1989). Alcohol and drug use also co-occur with Anxiety Disorders, Psychotic Disorders, and Personality Disorders in young people, and significantly complicate the diagnostic puzzle. It is prudent to assess carefully for other problems if there is a history of a Substance Use Disorder; at the same time, some caution is advised in diagnosis when a significant Substance Use Disorder occurs in apparent combination with other serious psychiatric disorders. In at least some cases, the clinical picture will change rather dramatically following a few months of sobriety and abstinence.

One specific word of warning applies to the diagnosis of comorbid Personality Disorders. Great caution is advised with respect to making Personality Disorder diagnoses in individuals who are in Early Partial or Full Remission from Substance Dependence, because this early period is apparently often characterized by interpersonal conflict and emotional lability, which could support a false-positive diagnosis of a Personality Disorder. Noting dysfunctional personality traits on Axis II (and treating them if necessary) is certainly useful and warranted however, a clinical assessment of Personality Disorders is often best delayed until after several months of Sustained Full Remission.

Use and misuse of substances tend to exacerbate a range of impulse control problems in adolescents. One particular area of concern regards an association between substance abuse and "risky" sexual behavior in adolescents (Langer & Tubman, 1997). Substance use and misuse are associated with unplanned pregnancies in teenage females.

Finally, the relationship between Substance Use Disorders and at least one Mental Disorder may vary with the client's gender. As discussed in Chapter 5, Posttraumatic Stress Disorder, (PTSD) may develop secondary to Substance Use Disorders in adolescent males, because substance use potentiates their interaction in and exposure to situations in which trauma is more likely. In adolescent females, however, Substance Use Disorders are often secondary to PTSD, possibly as a faulty coping response to the extreme emotional pain precipitated by the original trauma (Deykin & Buka, 1997).

Substance-Induced Disorders

Substance-Induced Disorders consist of a number of substance-specific patterns of maladjustment associated with a history of substance use. The two general syndromes identified are Substance Intoxication and Substance Withdrawal. In addition, various Substance-Induced Mental Disorders are found outside the "Substance-Related Disorders" chapter in DSM-IV (their placement is based on the type of behavioral symptoms elicited). These are listed on page 192 of the manual.

Differential Diagnosis

Substance Abuse and Dependence are significant mental health problems for many adolescents and children, and cases of Substance Intoxication and Withdrawal within the school setting are unfortunately all too familiar to most practicing school psychologists. The framework of DSM-IV's coverage of Substance-Related Disorders appears initially to be very confusing, because of the large numbers of discrete diagnoses covered and the similarity of several category titles; however, the apparent complexity reduces to four basic syndromes (plus a Not Otherwise Specified [NOS] category for each substance class) applied to 11 classes of substances, plus Other (or Unknown) and Polysubstance. With relatively little applied experience, the approach becomes familiar and relatively easy to use.

Another diagnostic difficulty is often harder to resolve: Substance use problems in youth have a high potential for pulling at the personal values and beliefs of the examiner in a way that is different from most mental health problems. Although there is probably wide-spread agreement among psychologists that depression is bad, learning to read is good, and being able to interact securely with one's social community is desirable, there is probably considerable ambivalence about what levels of illicit alcohol use, experimental smoking, and occasional use of "mild" hallucinogens (e.g., marijuana from a known supplier) are acceptable or tolerable among young, middle, and older adolescents. We appear unsure as a society of what our attitudes about substance use are or should be. Many professionals I interact with are troubled by the hypocrisy of a society that spends millions on alcohol and tobacco but tells its youth they should abstain. Some are bothered over the discrepancy between their own substance use (past or present) and the message society would like to convey to its young people. When a high school senior drinks a beer at a party occasionally, is this substance use or Substance Abuse? The answers are sometimes less than clear (Newcomb & Bentler, 1989).

I personally have come to operate with a low threshold for assessing the presence of substance use problems in youth. I tend to classify almost any recurrent or regular use of a controlled or illicit substance as problematic, any use of an inhalant as problematic, and any regular use of alcohol associated with complications of life as problematic. Among other considerations is the reality that obtaining these substances involves young persons in criminal behavior and usually brings them into associations with criminals. (If the circumstances do not justify a diagnosis of a Substance-Related Disorder, there are several potentially relevant V codes, including Child or Adolescent Antisocial Behavior.) My personal experience over a career focused largely on assessment of cognitive, emotional, and behavioral disorders has been that failure to assess aggressively for Substance Abuse and Dependence have accounted for the majority of my diagnostic errors. Use of both prescription and illicit drugs is widespread among youth in our society (Anthony, Warner, & Kessler, 1994) and clearly interacts with other personal and situational factors to affect adaptive behavior and overall functioning. Sensitivity to the general view of Substance Abuse and Dependence as conceptualized within DSM-IV, and review of the substance-specific features of intoxication and withdrawal reactions, can help increase examiners' alertness to signs of a potential Substance-Related Disorder and can prompt active investigation of relevant symptoms.

A related issue is the high comorbidity of substance use and misuse in youth with other mental disorders, as described above. Substance use problems appear often in the lives of young people preceding, during, and following the manifestation of other emotional and behavioral disturbances. Substance misuse exacerbates most of the other Mental Disorders discussed in this text. In my experience and judgment, substance use and Substance Use Disorders should always be part of the differential diagnosis in evaluating any older child or adolescent. Especially in any acutely developing problem in a young person without previous mental health problems, there should be a high index of suspicion regarding possible substance involvement.

Other Relevant Categories

Within the "Other Conditions That May Be a Focus of Clinical Attention" chapter are two sections related to medications. Medication-Induced Movement Disorders include several diagnoses of movement disorders associated with neuroleptic (antipsychotic) medications; however, these are seldom seen in children and adolescents. There is also the single diagnostic category Adverse Effects of Medication NOS, under the general heading of Other Medication-Induced Disorder. This condition, though not a Mental Disorder, should be noted on Axis I when the treatment of side effects from a medication becomes a main focus of treatment. For instance, exacerbation of tic problems in a child being treated for ADHD with a stimulant medication may become a therapy target; if so, the problem should be identified with this diagnosis.

OTHER "ADDICTIVE" BEHAVIORS

Various other behavior problems seem to have an "addictive" quality and have been conceptualized as behavioral analogues of Substance Use Disorders. The responsiveness of some of these behavior problems to the selective serotonin reuptake inhibitor (SSRI) antidepressant medications, and the advancement of the "dopamine hypothesis" regarding addictive behavior, have focused considerable attention on these problems and the issue they raise. Regardless of how they are ultimately understood, it is worth considering several of these problem behaviors.

Within the "Impulse-Control Disorders Not Elsewhere Classified" chapter are several diagnoses that have been informally described as "addictions." All of the diagnoses within this chapter of the manual have as their essential feature the failure to resist a drive, impulse, or temptation that the individual recognizes as harmful to self or others. Four of the diagnoses (Kleptomania, Pyromania, Pathological Gambling, and Trichotillomania) are characterized by active motivation to behave in a certain way. The fifth specific diagnosis (Intermittent Explosive Disorder) seems qualitatively different, in that it represents a failure to inhibit uncontrolled rage and aggression; this diagnosis has been discussed previously in Chapter 4. There is also a residual diagnosis: Impulse-Control Disorder NOS.

Kleptomania

Kleptomania can be an Impulse-Control Disorder, but the examiner should be highly cautious about regarding shoplifting among adolescents as Kleptomania. DSM-IV reports that Kleptomania is a rare condition among identified shoplifters (fewer than 5%). I am unaware of any empirical literature on Kleptomania among adolescents or children, and I have only seen a very few apparent cases of this disorder (all among teenagers). Shoplifting can occur either as an isolated delinquent act (Child or Adolescent Antisocial Behavior—a V code, not a Mental Disorder) or as part of the Conduct Disorder pattern. Shoplifting is also sometimes seen as a manifestation of Adjustment Disorder With Disturbance of Conduct. True Kleptomania, by contrast, appears to be primarily driven by tension reduction.

Pyromania

Pyromania does occur in adolescents, although rarely. There is often an erotic element in Pyromania, and this disorder may be more similar in some respects to the Paraphilias than to the other Impulse-Control Disorders (see Chapter 7). Fire-setting behavior is a concern in children and adolescents (DSM-IV reports that over 40% of individuals arrested for arson in the United States are under 18 years of age), but it is usually associated with Conduct Disorder, ADHD, Adjustment Disorder With Disturbance of Conduct, or Child or Adolescent Antisocial Behavior (which, again, is not a mental disorder).

Pathological Gambling

Pathological Gambling often begins during adolescence and sometimes during childhood. The refinement of the symptom criterion set from DSM-III through DSM-III-R to DSM-IV, and the development of psychometric instruments designed for the assessment of problematic teenage gambling (Shaffer, LaBrie, Scanlan, & Cummings, 1994),

should both bring needed attention to this often overlooked disturbance of youth.

Trichotillomania

Recurrent pulling out of one's own hair and failure to resist the impulse to pull one's hair, despite concern over the behavior and/or its
consequences (hair loss), define Trichotillomania. Associated behaviors often involve manipulation of the hair or, sometimes, eating the
hair ("trichophagia"). I believe that most cases of this may in fact be
variants of Obsessive–Compulsive Disorder (OCD), although there
has been only partial empirical support for this position (King et al.,
1995). Conceptually, the absence of an obsession in Trichotillomania
should distinguish between the two diagnoses, but I find that this
differentiation often breaks down in actual clinical cases. The matter
is further complicated by the comorbidities between this behavior
and Mood Disorders, Anxiety Disorders (including OCD), and Mental Retardation, as well as by the mutual positive response reported
for OCD and Trichotillomania to the SSRI antidepressants. King et
al. (1995) note that children with Trichotillomania often do not report rising tension of relief with hair pulling, which is at odds with
the common experience of individuals with an Impulse-Control Disorder. It is probably worthwhile diagnosing this specific pattern of
compulsive behavior to ensure that it is specifically targeted for treatment.

Impulse-Control Disorder Not Otherwise Specified

The residual category of Impulse-Control Disorder NOS can be used
to classify other repetitive patterns of self-limiting or self-destructive
behavior that have a driven quality of failure to resist an impulse.
Fisher (1994) has developed a proposed criterion set, modeled on
the DSM-IV diagnosis of Pathological Gambling, for "video game addiction" in children and adolescents. Gupta and Derevensky (1996)
have discussed similarities between video games and gambling activities.

HARMFUL ENVIRONMENTAL EFFECTS

In addition to intentional exposure to the chemical effects of alcohol
and other drugs, exposure to a variety of other deleterious environ-

mental forces can play a role in the origins of and forms taken by cognitive, behavioral, and emotional problems. The role of a "toxic" environment has received a great deal of attention in the effort to understand child and adolescent maladjustment. Whether harmful environmental factors are emotional or physical (or chemical) the short- and long-term effects of experiential adversity are of growing concern among mental health workers. Although categories for different forms of child maltreatment have been available for some time within ICD-9-CM, it was not until the publication of DSM-IV that V codes involving abuse and neglect were provided for within the DSM system. These (and other) deleterious environmental effects are considered in the "Other Conditions That May Be a Focus of Clinical Attention" chapter. As noted throughout this book, these are not Mental Disorders but may be of critical importance. In addition, I discuss one mental disorder here that involves disturbed parenting or caretaking.

Reactive Attachment Disorder of Infancy or Early Childhood

Reactive Attachment Disorder of Infancy or Early Childhood (abbreviated here as RAD) is an Axis I Mental Disorder from the "Disorders Usually First Diagnosed in Infancy, Childhood, or Adolescence" chapter. This disturbance consists essentially of inappropriate social relatedness and attachment between a young child and parent or primary caretaker because of "grossly pathological care" (p. 116). Attention is given in the diagnostic criteria to providing an objective definition of "pathological care." This disorder has two subtypes: an Inhibited Type, in which there is a failure to initiate or respond to social interactions as expected; and a Disinhibited Type, in which the child shows indiscriminate sociability and lack of differential responsiveness. RAD may occur in association with eating problems (Feeding Disorder of Infancy or Early Childhood, Pica, Rumination Disorder) and developmental delays, as well as with the V codes of Physical Abuse of Child, Sexual Abuse of Child, Neglect of Child, and Parent–Child Relational Problem. The differentiation between RAD and Pervasive Developmental Disorders (which also show deviant social responsiveness and attachment) is based on the usual availability in the latter of supportive social environments, as well as on the additional symptom clusters seen in Pervasive Developmental Disorders.

Boris, Zeanah, Larrieu, Scheeringa, and Heller (1998) have recently raised a serious challenge regarding the reliability of the DSM-IV diagnostic criteria for RAD, and have proposed alternative criteria with acceptable reliability. As these authors state, their results need to

be replicated. As for the practicing school or child psychologist concerned with potential cases of RAD, it is the responsibility of the evaluator to indicate clearly whether any alternative diagnostic criteria have
been employed in clinical decision making. One possible course of
action may be to employ both the DSM-IV and the proposed alternative criteria of Boris and his coinvestigators. Where both sets agree
(on either the presence or absence of characteristics), the examiner
can feel confident in his or her diagnostic conclusions. Disagreement
between the two sets may indicate a need for further evaluation.

Physical Abuse of Child, Sexual Abuse of Child, and Neglect of Child

Three categories from the "Other Conditions That May Be a Focus of
Clinical Attention" chapter identify deviant behavior toward a child
(or adolescent): Neglect of Child, Physical Abuse of Child, and Sexual
Abuse of Child. The ICD-9-CM codes for these patterns of destructive
involvement with a young person differ, depending on who is the
focus of clinical attention—the abused or neglected youth, or the
perpetrator. The next Coding Note describes these different codes,
and also notes recent changes in the codes used when the young victim is the focus of attention. The decision not to classify these three
behavior patterns as mental disorders appears consistent with the
overarching view of troubled actions versus Mental Disorders adhered
to by DSM-IV.

CODING NOTE   Child Maltreatment

Physical Abuse of Child, Sexual Abuse of Child, and Neglect of Child
receive different ICD-9 CM codes, depending on whether the focus of
clinical attention is on the young victim of malteatment or on the
dysfunctional caretaker. In cases where the focus is on the caretaker,
the same code (V61.21) is used for all three conditions. A single code
number (995.5) was originally also used in cases focusing on the young
victim. However, with the recent changes in coding referred to earlier
in the Coding Notes on pp. 49 and 92 (see American Psychiatric Association, 1996a, 1996b), these conditions now receive separate ICD-9-
CM codes in such cases:

995.54   Physical Abuse of Child
995.53   Sexual Abuse of Child
995.52   Neglect of Child

♦♦♦

Highly Focused
Symptom Patterns

♦

A number of behavior problems commonly seen in children and adolescents revolve around single symptoms or very circumscribed problem areas. Historically, difficulties with eating, sleep, elimination,
movement, and speech, and other focused disturbances of functioning, were discussed as "habit problems." In DSM-II these were grouped
in a section titled "Special Symptoms." From DSM-III onward, this
heterogeneous grouping has been divided among several categories:
Several are addressed in the "Disorders Usually First Diagnosed in
Infancy, Childhood, or Adolescence" chapter, whereas other are addressed in chapters covering specific problem areas (e.g., Sleep Disorders, Eating Disorders). Among the more commonly seen of these
symptom patterns in school-age children are eating, elimination, and
sleep problems. I discuss these in this chapter, along with tics, sexual
and gender identity problems, and a few others. They are presented
in the order in which the first problem in each group appears in DSM-
IV.

EATING PROBLEMS

When disturbances of eating behavior, diet, and weight are being evaluated, three different areas of DSM-IV need to be considered: the "Feeding and Eating Disorders of Infancy or Early Childhood" section in
the "Disorders Usually First Diagnosed in Infancy, Childhood, or
Adolescence" chapter (pp. 94–100); the "Eating Disorders" chapter

(pp. 539–550), and the description of Psychological Factors Affecting Medical Condition in the "Other Conditions That May Be a Focus of Clinical Attention" chapter (pp. 675–678). If the reader finds this arrangement confusing, that is because it is an awkward and confusing arrangement. DSM-V may provide a more coherent or at least a simpler arrangement, but for the present it is necessary to remember that eating problems may be described at several places in the text. In an alternative view of this arrangement, Kerwin and Berkowitz (1996) cite as an advantage of DSM-IV as the reclassification of ingestive problems into two broad groupings (Feeding and Eating Disorders of Infancy or Early Childhood, and Eating Disorders). Kerwin and Berkowitz believe this arrangement to be consistent with data indicating that these two groupings reflect different populations and have no evidence of continuity between them. This is certainly the case but given the thematic arrangement of DSM-IV seemly hardly to justify independent placement. Furthermore, the logic of Kerwin and Berkowitz appears to imply greater homogeneity within these two broad groupings than can be supported on the basis of the empirical literature.

Specific eating behaviors (symptoms) may occur as primary or associated symptoms of several mental disorders. For example, significant weight loss or gain and/or decrease or increase in appetite can be a symptom of Major Depressive Disorder, Dysthymic Disorder, or Depressive Disorder Not Otherwise Specified (NOS); appetite loss can occur in the context of Generalized Anxiety Disorder; and food rituals may develop in the course of Obsessive–Compulsive Disorder (OCD) or Schizophrenia). However, when one primary focus of clinical attention becomes a recurrent pattern of difficulty involving food consumption and diet, an eating-related mental disorder should be considered. Feeding and Eating Disorders of Infancy or Early Childhood occur by definition in relatively young populations. Eating Disorders tend to occur most frequently in adolescence, but with some significant incidence during childhood (and adult life). For clients of all ages, the association of eating problems with physiological problems and medical instability should be kept in mind (Palla & Litt, 1988).

Feeding and Eating Disorders of Infancy or Early Childhood

Three specific diagnoses of eating behavior remain in the first content chapter of DSM-IV (which, as stressed throughout this book, should not be referred to as the "child section"): Pica, Rumination Disorder, and Feeding Disorder of Infancy or Early Childhood.

PICA

Pica is the consistent consumption of nonnutritive substances for at least a 1-month period. "Scavenging behavior" is an alternative phrase occasionally used in the literature to describe eating nonfood substances. Historically, the nosological practice was to identify the substance eaten (e.g., "geophagia," eating clays or other earthy substances; "coprophagia," eating feces; "trichophagia," eating hair). Occasional mouthing, chewing, or eating of nonnutritive substances is not uncommon during the first 2 years of life and should not be diagnosed as Pica unless the behavior is problematic. Pica appears to be more common in developmentally delayed populations, and may be more common in environments with limited stimulation. A major concern in cases of Pica is the risk of poisoning, especially exposure to lead, which is highly toxic. Pica can occur as an associated symptom of broad patterns of maladjustment (e.g., Pervasive Developmental Disorders or Schizophrenia) or of neurological disorders (e.g., Kleine–Levin syndrome. In these cases, a separate diagnosis of Pica should only be made if the eating disturbance is serious enough to require formal clinical attention (a treatment plan, behavior modification program, or similar therapy focus).

Rumination Disorder

Rumination Disorder involves the persistent regurgitation and rechewing of food, typically in an infant or very young child. It occurs after a period of normal eating behavior and goes on for at least a month. There is often an association with general developmental delays. If there is an associated Pervasive Developmental Disorder or Mental Retardation, Rumination Disorder should only be independently diagnosed if it warrants focused treatment. Rumination during the course of Anorexia Nervosa or Bulimia Nervosa (see Eating Disorders below) are not separately diagnosed.

Feeding Disorder of Infancy or Early Childhood

Feeding Disorder of Infancy or Early Childhood reflects a nonorganic failure to thrive for at least a 1-month period before a child reaches age 6. Careful medical evaluation is necessary to rule out biological causes. When primary organic causes have been excluded, the possible contributing factors include infant characteristics which may make caretaking difficult, as well as inadequate skills and knowledge or maladjustment on the part of the caretaker(s). Again, the problems must begin during the first 6 years of life.

Eating Disorders

Three disorders are included in the "Eating Disorders" chapter: Anorexia Nervosa (AN), Bulimia Nervosa (BN), and Eating Disorder
NOS (see the next IDEA Note). The most useful categorization of
Eating Disorders in adolescents and adults, and the boundaries between these syndromes, continue to be actively investigated areas. Longitudinal studies continue to underscore the complexity of patterns
of dysfunctional eating behavior, as well as the multiple associations
with other patterns of emotional and behavioral maladjustment (Hall,
Slim, Hawker, & Salmond, 1984).

Anorexia Nervosa

AN reflects a loss of normal weight (or failure to gain expected weight
over time) associated with a morbid fear of being obese, a perceptual
disturbance in body image, and (in postmenarcheal females) amen-
orrhea (i.e., cessation of menstrual periods). AN is one of the few
mental disorders with greater female than male prevalence; the majority of cases are females. Onset of clinical AN is often in adolescence, but concerns with body image and weight often develop prior
to puberty (Sands, Tricker, Sherman, Armatas, & Maschette, 1997).
DSM-IV points out that the term "anorexia" (loss of appetite) is usually a misnomer; most women with AN do not report loss of appetite,
but rather a much more powerful fear of gaining excessive weight.
The popular image of the client with AN as relying on self-induced
vomiting (the "two finger restroom run") is also not completely accurate. Some individuals with AN do make use of "purging behavior"—
self-induced vomiting and/or abuse of emetics, laxatives, diuretics,

---

IDEA NOTE   Eating Disorders and IDEA

Eating problems seem to be frequent in older children and adolescents in our society, and surveys often report disturbing prevalence
rates of eating disturbances that could be classified as an Eating Disorder Not Otherwise Specified (Steiner & Lock, 1998). Despite this prevalence, however, eating problems come directly to the attention of school
psychologists relatively rarely. I have seldom seen the issue of an eating
disorder addressed in an Individual Educational Plan. Nevertheless,
eating disorders would appear to be covered under the "seriously emotionally disturbed" IDEA category. The rationale and documentation
would be similar to that used for Mood Disorders (see the IDEA Note
on p. 78).

---

or enemas. As common or more common in my experience is the more prosaic behavior of restricting eating excessively, sometimes in association with high-frequency/long-duration exercise. What clinically identifies the young person with AN is a body weight below normal.

Strong associations are reported between AN and current or future Major Depressive Episodes, and I would recommend a careful assessment of possible mood disturbance or Mood Disorders in a young person with an Eating Disorder. Suicide is one factor contributing to the mortality associated with AN, and suicide risk should be carefully evaluated. Both because of the medical complications associated with starvation (as well as purging behavior, if this occurs) and because of the risk of suicide, AN is a life-threatening mental disorder, and an identified case requires aggressive treatment. In older adolescents and adults with AN, there may also be comorbid personality trait disturbances or Personality Disorders. OCD and Obsessive–Compulsive Personality Disorder may be overrepresented in patients with AN (Thornton & Russell, 1997).

Although AN is usually discussed in terms of a female clinical population, it is necessary to keep in mind that 5–10% of reported cases are male. Furthermore, the proportion of males may increase in childhood-onset cases (Bryant-Waugh & Lask, 1995). The DSM-IV criterion set for AN has some inherent limitations for males and premenarcheal females. Alternative diagnostic criteria have been suggested (Bryant-Waugh & Lask, 1995) to deal with these and other assessment issues, but the examiner needs to make it very clear whether a diagnosis is being based on DSM-IV or an alternative set of criteria.

Bulimia Nervosa

BN is a pattern of disturbance in which the individual (again, usually female), though excessively concerned with the body weight and shape, experiences periods of loss of control over eating. Huge quantities of various foods, often high-calorie foods, are consumed. Despite these "binge" episodes, the young woman maintains a normal body weight. Maintaining a stable weight despite periodic ferocious overconsumption requires a compensatory mechanism to rid the body of the excessive calories consumed; this is the "purge" half of the binge–purge cycle of BN. Self-induced vomiting; abuse of emetics, diuretics, laxatives, and/or enemas; excessive exercise; and total fasting may be used singly or in various combinations to discard the excessive calories consumed during the binge. BN behaviors, especially the compensatory mechanisms used, are medically dangerous. One factor contributing to the mortality of BN (as well as that of AN when purging is involved) is sudden coronary arrest associated with the electrolyte imbalances caused by purging. Among the medical morbidities, serious dental problems associated with recurrent vomiting are frequently seen.

Behavioral problems frequently found in association with BN include depression and suicidal behavior, as well as self-injurious behavior. Greater substance use has been found in adolescents with bulimic behavior, and the combination of BN and increased substance use predicts impulsive acting out in female adolescents—attempted suicide, stealing, and sexual activity (Wiederman & Pryor, 1996). Personality Disorders may be more commonly associated with BN than with AN, and a comorbid diagnosis of Borderline Personality Disorder should be ruled out. Like, BN is a potentially life-threatening disorder. The clinical situation is complicated by the normal appearance of the young person, which impedes identification of this deadly pattern of maladjustment. In childhood-onset BN, associated problems of depression and poor self-image are reported (Bryant-Waugh & Lask, 1995).

Eating Disorder Not Otherwise Specified

The residual category of Eating Disorder NOS is used for clinical cases that do not meet the full criteria for a specific Eating Disorder or show other atypical patterns of eating. Eating Disorder NOS may be especially helpful in work with children: Bryant-Waugh and Lask (1995) found that 25% of referrals to an eating disorders clinic were not well classified by DSM-IV. The atypical patterns they found included "food avoidance emotional disorder," "selective eating," and "pervasive refusal syndrome" (Bryant-Waugh & Lask, 1995). One of the categories proposed for further study in Appendix B of DSM-IV is Binge-Eating Disorder (pp. 729–731). Binge-Eating Disorder is a pattern of abnormal consumption, loss of usual sense of choice or control over eating, and distress; without the dangerous compensatory behaviors of BN. Binge-Eating Disorder would currently be diagnosed as Eating Disorder NOS.

Psychological Factors Affecting Medical Condition

A final category relevant to eating problems, that of Psychological Factors Affecting Medical Condition, can be used to describe cases where emotional and behavioral difficulties contribute to overeating. Obesity is included in ICD-9-CM as a general medical condition, but simple overeating is not identified as a mental disorder in DSM-IV. If there is convincing evidence that psychological factors play a significant role in a case of obesity, this can be reflected by a notation of

Maladaptive Health Behaviors Affecting Obesity. (Maladaptive Health Behaviors Affecting . . . is one of the specific conditions included under Psychological Factors Affecting Medical Condition.)

TIC DISORDERS

Four diagnoses are provided for the classification of Tic Disorders: Tourette's Disorder, Chronic Motor or Vocal Tic Disorder, Transient Tic Disorder, and Tic Disorder NOS. Broadly described, these categories represent various combinations of tic pattern (vocal and/or motor) and duration (less than or more than 1 year). All but Tic Disorder NOS require an onset prior to 18 years of age. Tourette's Disorder involves both motor and vocal tics and a prolonged duration; Chronic Motor or Vocal Tic Disorder reflects either motor or vocal tics and a prolonged duration; Transient Tic Disorder covers any pattern that has caused difficulty for at least 4 weeks but less than 1 year; and Tic Disorder NOS covers problems during the first month, as well as problems with onset after the age of 18. A great deal of psychological interest has focused on Tourette's Disorder and on the possibility of a spectrum of neurobehavioral disorders that includes many Tic Disorders, OCD, and Attention-Deficit/Hyperactivity Disorder (ADHD). There are significant comorbidities between Tourette's Disorder and OCD, as well as between Tourette's Disorder and ADHD. Walter and Carter (1997) suggest that learning problems are also overrepresented in children with Tourette's Disorder, although most do not have learning or cognitive disabilities. Children who present with Tic Disorders should be periodically evaluated for attention deficit problems as well as anxiety symptoms, especially obsessive–compulsive patterns.

ELIMINATION DISORDERS

DSM-IV provides for the diagnosis of two Elimination Disorders: Encopresis and Enuresis. There is no provision for atypical presentations or cases that do not meet the criteria for the two categories (e.g., frequent urinary incontinence in a 4-year-old with average intelligence, leading to marked family conflict, emotional distress on the part of the child, and disruption of peer relationships and adjustment). The criterion sets presented are clear and take cognizance of the functional distinctions supported by the empirical literature with respect to frequency of incidents, age of onset, diurnal–nocturnal pattern, and history of continence.

It needs to be stressed that Enuresis is, by definition, not caused by disease or structural abnormality (cases of organic incontinence); the full title in DSM-IV is Enuresis (Not Due to a General Medical Condition). While research into the etiology of "primary course" (no history of established urinary continence) Nocturnal Only Enuresis strongly suggests that it does have a biological basis, it is distinct from urinary incontinence associated with infections and systemic illnesses. Both Enuresis and incontinence will come to the attention of teachers and school psychologists. It is important to ensure that a proper medical evaluation has ruled out possible organic causes. Apparent "Enuresis" may be an early symptom of juvenile-onset diabetes, as well as of sickle cell anemia or related disorders. Although cases of organic urinary incontinence in children are rare (some estimates suggest that as few as 5% of all cases of voiding of urine into bed or clothes involve illness or structural abnormalities), ensuring that these cases are accurately identified and treated is a responsibility of all professionals involved with children.

MISCELLANEOUS SYMPTOM PATTERNS

Selective Mutism

Selective Mutism (Elective Mutism in DSM-III and DSM-III-R) has also been referred to as "voluntary silence." This is an interesting pattern that may manifest itself primarily in the school setting. The child in question is able to talk (documented by observation in other settings) but chooses not to in at least one specific social setting, causing social or educational problems. Although Selective Mutism is often discussed in the context of communication difficulties, approximately two-thirds of children with the disorder Mutism have no other unusual speech characteristics. The problem appears to be more of a behavioral disturbance than a communication difficulty. This view is supported by a recent study by Dummit et al. (1997), which finds that Selective Mutism usually presents in the context of Anxiety Disorders. Steinhausen and Juzi (1996) reported that shyness and internalizing behavior problems were the most frequent personality features noted in a series of 100 cases of DSM-III-R Elective Mutism. Selective Mutism may be comorbid with Social Phobia, and both disorders should be diagnosed in such a case. A population study covering two school districts in Sweden found a higher prevalence rate than had been previously estimated—approximately 18 cases per 10,000 children aged 7–15 years (Kopp & Gillberg, 1997). The association of Selective Mutism with social reticence, possibly in the parents as well as the child, may act to suppress detection and awareness of this problem (Kopp & Gillberg, 1997).

Stereotypic Movement Disorder

Stereotypic Movement Disorder (Atypical Stereotyped Movement Disorder in DSM-III, Stereotypy/Habit Disorder in DSM-III-R) consists of repetitive, nonpurposeful motor movements that have a "driven" quality. The actions may be self-injurious, in which case the specifier With Self-Injurious Behavior is added to the diagnosis. This type of behavior is a common associated feature of Pervasive Developmental Disorders, and the diagnosis of Stereotypic Movement Disorder is not made concurrently with a diagnosis of such a disorder. Stereotypic Movement Disorder may also be associated with Mental Retardation, and the diagnosis can be made concurrently with that of Mental Retardation if the stereotypic or self-injurious actions are problematic enough to warrant a treatment focus.

SEXUAL AND GENDER IDENTITY DISORDERS

As its title indicates, the "Sexual and Gender Identity Disorders" chapter of DSM-IV discusses three groups of problems unified by some issue of human sexuality or gender; there is also a residual classification, Sexual Disorder NOS. Sexual Dysfunctions have limited application in school psychology and are relatively clearly presented. Paraphilias become matters of concern in adolescence, and Gender Identity Disorders may come to clinical attention at any age.

Paraphilias reflect deviant sexual arousal, urges, or behavior. Several classical patterns (Exhibitionism, Fetishism, Frotteurism, Pedophilia, Sexual Masochism, Sexual Sadism, Transvestic Fetishism, and Voyeurism) are specified in DSM-IV, and a residual category (Paraphilia NOS) is provided for less common patterns (telephone scatologia, necrophilia, zoophilia, coprophilia, klismaphilia, and urophilia, to mention only a few). It is worth reiterating that the diagnosis of a mental disorder refers typically to a pattern of behavior (not an isolated act) that has significant functional consequences (clinically relevant distress or impairment). Occasionally a psychologist is consulted by a teenager concerned that "a friend" has had a dream that included disturbing sexual behavior. Whatever their therapeutic uses, dream content is not the basis upon which Paraphilias are diagnosed—much to the relief, usually, of the teenager involved. Wulfert, Greenway, and Dougher (1996) have drawn interesting parallels between Pedophilia and alcoholism, based on a functional analysis of "reinforcement-based disorders."

Gender Identity Disorder reflects a basic conflict between individuals' sense of themselves as males, females, or persons of ambivalent gender on the one hand, and their assigned sex on the other. Coding is based on the age of the client; Gender Identity Disorder in

Children and Gender Identity Disorder in Adolescents or Adults have different ICD-9-CM codes. There is also a Gender Identity Disorder NOS category to cover a very heterogeneous group of residual problems involving gender identity elements. These disorders will be rare in the experience of most school and child clinical psychologists. Multiple clinical and social issues are raised by both psychological and medical treatments of gender identity problems (Nordyke, Baer, Etzel, & LeBlanc, 1977; Rekers & Lovaas, 1974; Wolfe, 1979; Zucker, 1990). Beyond initial identification, a referral to a specialized assessment facility is usually the most appropriate disposition (Cohen-Kettenis & van Goozen, 1997). In working with youth with Gender Identity Disorder, it is useful to be aware of this disorder's association with symptoms of internalizing behavior problems and with Separation Anxiety Disorder (see Bradley & Zucker, 1997). The next IDEA Note sets forth how Gender Identity Disorder relates to eligibility for services under IDEA.

SLEEP DISORDERS

Sleep problems are probably common in children, but are not often the basis of psychological evaluations. DSM-IV distinguishes four major groups: Primary Sleep Disorders, Sleep Disorder Related to Another Mental Disorder, Sleep Disorder Due to a General Medical Condition, and Substance-Induced Sleep Disorder. The Primary Sleep Disorders are further subdivided into Dyssomnias (problems with the quality, amount, or timing of sleep) and Parasomnias (abnormal behavior in association with sleep, sleep stages, or transitions).

IDEA NOTE   Gender Identity Disorder and IDEA

Gender Identity Disorder is a highly specific and infrequent pattern of maladjustment in youth and is not found on the list of qualifying conditions for special education or other special services in IDEA. However, diagnosis may qualify for inclusion under IDEA for services through the "seriously mentally disturbed" category. Both the short- and long-term consequences of Gender Identity Disorder are severe and negative, especially for males. Young females may find their peers and adult caretakers more tolerant of their violation of sex role behavior, but young males tend to meet with harsh rejection and social abuse. The impact of ostracism and isolation on their social development can be profound and long-lasting, extending into their social adjustment as adults.

A valuable addition to the text of DSM-IV is a section under each Sleep Disorder category that relates the DSM-IV categories to those in *The International Classification of Sleep Disorders: Diagnostic and Coding Manual* (ICSD). This classification was published by the American Sleep Disorders Association (1990) and is an important reference for investigators and clinicians specializing in Sleep Disorders. The ICSD has recently been revised and republished (American Sleep Disorders Association, 1997), so some of the correspondences have altered, but the effort to relate DSM-IV to other influential documents in specialized areas has been an important step forward.

Sleep problems that occur in association with other mental disorders are seen with some regularity in clinical practice, especially in the context of Mood or Anxiety Disorders. The independent diagnosis of Sleep Disorder Related to Another Mental Disorder is only made when the sleep problem is severe enough to warrant being a focus of treatment. The same stipulation applies to Sleep Disorder Due to a General Medical Condition and Substance-Induced Sleep Disorder.

A related phenomenon is "bruxism" (teeth grinding). Nocturnal bruxism is often considered under the general heading of sleep problems. In an informative review article, Glaros and Melamed (1992) offer the following definition: "Bruxism is the nonfunctional contact of the teeth, including clenching, gnashing, grinding, and tapping" (p. 192). Bruxism is usually of concern because of potential dental damage rather than worry over a child's or adolescent's psychological adjustment. Despite interest in stress as a contributing factor, the literature in general does not suggest mental disorders in most children who grind their teeth (Glaros & Melamed, 1992). Bruxism is identified as a mental disorder in ICD-9-CM (306.8, "Other specified psychophysiological malfunction, Bruxism, Teeth grinding"), but it is not included in DSM-IV. Nocturnal teeth grinding can be coded as Sleep Disorder NOS. Diurnal bruxism can be recorded on Axis III if the sole concern is dental. Diurnal bruxism in which stress and emotional adjustment are significant factors can also be coded on Axis I under Psychological Factors Affecting Medical Condition (and the bruxism can be noted on Axis III). The case of bruxism illustrates the general point that while all DSM-IV diagnostic categories have legitimate ICD-9-CM diagnostic codes, the converse is not true. Several mental health and medical conditions are risk factors for bruxism—cerebral palsy, Mental Retardation in general, trisomy 21 (Down's Syndrome) in particular, and treatment with stimulant medications (Glaros & Melamed, 1992).

◆

See DSM-IV-TR Coding Notes: Tic Disorders in DSM-IV-TR, Stereotypic Movement Disorder in DSM-IV-TR, and Sexual Disorders in DSM-IV-TR, in 2002 Updates, pages 235–236.

CHAPTER 8

♦♦♦

Problems with Mental Ability, Learning, Communication, and Cognition

♦

OVERVIEW

Problems with mental ability, learning, communication, and cognition receive primary focus in DSM-IV in four areas: Mental Retardation; Learning Disorders; Communication Disorders; and Delirium Dementia, and Amnestic and Other Cognitive Disorders. (Two V codes, Borderline Intellectual Functioning and Academic Problem, may also be applicable in some cases.) The first three areas are found the "Disorders Usually First Diagnosed in Infancy, Childhood, or Adolescence" chapter, whereas the fourth is covered in a separate chapter dealing with what were previously known as Organic Mental Disorders. The school psychologist is well prepared to assess children with respect to the first three areas, although many may find the diagnoses available for learning problems within DSM-IV less than satisfying. The use of the diagnoses for cognitive problems in DSM-IV may be one of the greatest "stretches" for the practicing school psychologist.

It is worth recognizing that these are the only areas in DSM-IV where formal psychological or language assessment is mentioned or called for. Yet even here, the emphasis remains on the clinical assessment and judgment of the examiner. Formal testing may set limits within which judgment takes place, but it does not replace or supplant the primary responsibility of the examiner in determining the most appropriate diagnostic classification. Independent of its other strengths or weaknesses, DSM-IV is about assessment and not testing.

MENTAL RETARDATION AND RELATED PROBLEMS

Definitions and Subclassification of Mental Retardation

Little discussion of Mental Retardation (MR) with regard to making a DSM-IV diagnosis will be necessary. The school psychologist will find that the conceptualization of MR in DSM-IV is quite familiar, because it is based on the original tripartite conception of the former American Association on Mental Deficiency (Grossman, 1983; Heber, 1959, 1961): subnormal intellectual functioning, impairment in adaptive behavior, and onset during childhood or adolescence. The subclassification of MR in DSM-IV is based solely on the severity of intellectual impairment (tested IQ; see the following Application Note). In response to the most recently revised definition of MR by the American Association of Mental Retardation (AAMR, 1992), DSM-IV provides some discussion of the standard error of IQs and explicit acknowledgment of the possibility of a diagnosis of MR in an individual with a tested IQ between 70 and 75 *and* significant impairment in adaptive behaviors (see the following Professional Note). As in DSM-

---

APPLICATION NOTE   DSM-IV Subclassification of MR:
  Degrees of Severity

The DSM-IV subclassification of MR is based on level of tested intellectual ability and identifies four specific groups (plus the MR, Severity Unspecified category, for individuals whose intelligence cannot be validly assessed):

Mild MR	Tested IQ ranging from 50–55 to approximately 70
Moderate MR	Tested IQ ranging from 35–40 to 50–55
Severe MR	Tested IQ ranging from 20–25 to 35–40
Profound MR	Tested IQ below 20–25

A fuller view of the view of generalized cognitive limitations taken by DSM-IV is obtained by considering that a related category, Borderline Intellectual Functioning, extends the categorization to five diagnoses:

Borderline Intellectual Functioning	Tested IQ 71–84
Mild MR	Tested IQ ranging from 50–55 to approximately 70
Moderate MR	Tested IQ ranging from 35–40 to 50–55
Severe MR	Tested IQ 20–25 to 35–40
Profound MR	Tested IQ below 20–25

PROFESSIONAL NOTE   MR as Defined by DSM-IV and the AAMR

Despite similarities in the broad requirements, there are both conceptual and specific differences between the definition of MR in DSM-IV and that offered by the AAMR (1992) in the fourth revision of its seminal statement on diagnosis and classification of MR. A careful contrast of these two perspectives is beyond the purview of this work, but the school psychologist should consider carefully the argued advantages and disadvantages of both positions (Gresham, MacMillan, & Siperstein, 1995; Hodapp, 1995; MacMillan, Gresham, & Siperstein, 1993; Matson, 1995; Reiss, 1994a). The AAMR (1992) definition of MR retains the three basic elements articulated in the previoius original formulation (Grossman, 1983): significant subaverage intellectual functioning, related limitations in adaptive skill areas, and onset before age 18. Relative to previous editions, however, an even greater emphasis is placed on deficits in adaptive behavior; there is greater consideration of how the standard error of intelligence tests creates fuzzy boundaries at the limits of MR; and subclassification is based on the intensity of supports needed to support maximum adaptation in individuals with MR.

The practical implications of these seemingly subtle shifts of emphasis are potentially very significant. Greater attention to adaptive behavior creates an even greater need for valid and reliable measures of this important domain of adjustment. The possibility that an individual with a tested IQ between 70 and 75 (and clinically significant impairment in adaptive behavior) might be classified as having MR could potentially affect the official classification of a vast population of citizens. Basing the subclassification of MR on level of support rather than tested intelligence not only is a fundamental shift away from the standard practice of all previous classification system, but demands a methodology that has not yet been established as reliable or valid. Although DSM-IV has shown some response to the AAMR (1992) document in its increased discussion of the importance of adaptive behavior and the practical impact of the standard error of intelligence tests, the basic form of DSM-IV's conceptualization of MR has not been altered to match the new AAMR definition.

III-R, the four degrees of MR severity are given fuzzy boundaries. The adaptive behavior criterion has been made more detailed—it now explicitly considers 11 areas (see the next Application Note) and requires deficits or impaired effectiveness in 2 of these—but determination of these deficits is left up to the judgment of the examiner. The school psychologist should note that DSM-IV sets the age-of-origin

---

**APPLICATION NOTE   Areas of Adaptive Functioning
Considered with Regard to MR in DSM-IV**

Communication

Self-care

Home living

Social/interpersonal skills

Use of community resources

Self-direction

Functional academic skills

Work

Leisure

Health

Safety

---

criterion below age 18, in contrast to some alternative standards common in school settings. Finally, MR is one of the only two groups of mental disorder diagnoses coded on Axis II; the other group is the Personality Disorders (see the next Coding Note).

In addition to the four subcategories of MR defined by tested IQ

CODING NOTE   Avoiding a Common Error in Using DSM-IV

The MR diagnoses and the V code Borderline Intellectual Functioning are coded on Axis II. These diagnoses and the Personality Disorder diagnoses are the *only* diagnoses coded on Axis II in DSM-IV. Misplacement of MR and especially of Borderline Intellectual Functioning is an error commonly seen.

In DSM-III, Mental Retardation was coded on Axis I. Only the Specific Developmental Disorders (learning, language, and some speech disorders) and Personality Disorders were coded on Axis II.

In DSM-III-R, MR was moved to Axis II, along with the V code Borderline Intellectual functioning and the Pervasive Developmental Disorders. The Specific Developmental Disorders (now including the subgroups "Academic Skills Disorders, Language and Speech Disorders, and Motor Skill Disorders) and Personality Disorders remained on Axis II.

In DSM-IV, MR has been left on Axis II, along with Borderline Intellectual Functioning and Personality Disorders. The Pervasive Developmental Disorders, Learning Disorders, Motor Skills Disorder, and Communication Disorders have been returned to Axis I. Only the Personality Disorders have consistently remained on Axis II across the three presentations of DSM as a multiaxial diagnostic system.

---

levels, two other categories need to be considered: MR, Severity Unspecified, and Borderline Intellectual Functioning (see below).

It is worth considering that advances in understanding the genetic, physiological, and neurological bases of MR may finally result in improved clarity in our views of this large and highly heterogeneous population (see State, King, & Dykens, 1997). In their recent review, King, State, Shah, Davanzo, and Dykens (1997) note that MR "ranks first among chronic conditions that cause major limitations in activity for persons in the United States (Centers for Disease Control [and Prevention], 1996)" (p. 1662). Staying abreast of these developments will be one of the exciting challenges for school and clinical psychologists as the 21st century begins. The next IDEA Note sets forth how MR relates to eligibility for services under IDEA, and the following Professional Note discusses how MR relates to expectations for educability.

Mental Retardation, Severity Unspecified

MR, Severity Unspecified is used to cover cases where there is strong presumptive evidence of MR, but an acceptable measure of intellectual functioning is not available (the client cannot be tested, is uncooperative, or is otherwise impossible to assess). The availability of this diagnosis both gives DSM-IV considerable flexibility and challenges

---

IDEA NOTE   MR and IDEA

MR is an identified qualifying condition for special services under IDEA. This apparently straightforward statement is complicated, however, by variation in the meaning of "mental retardation" across the various documents and practices. The children identified by various state definitions as showing subaverage general intelligence may or may not qualify for a DSM-IV diagnosis of MR, which is a mental disorder. Children showing tested intellectual functioning in the range of 71 to 84 are assigned the DSM-IV V code of Borderline Intellectual Functioning, which is not a mental disorder category. Some of these children, especially these at the lower end of the range, will probably qualify for special services under the IDEA classification of "mental retardation." The situation is further confused by the apparent tendency of some school districts to classify some children who show the general pattern of Mild MR under the alternative conceptualization of "learning-disabled" (MacMillan, Gresham, Siperstein, & Bocian, 1996).

PROFESSIONAL NOTE   MR and Educability Expectations

The only serious competition to the traditional five-category model of "mental retardation" in psychiatry (borderline, mild, moderate, severe, profound) was the three-category model (educable, trainable, custodial), which evolved in education to help set educability expectations for mentally handicapped children. The original purpose of this diagnostic system was to establish responsibility for care. Prior to the passage of P.L. 94-142, many children classified as trainable and probably all classified as custodial were excluded from a free public education. P.L. 94-142 (and IDEA, which supplanted it) redefined the term "education" from a narrow focus on academic skills to a broader conception that included the development of adaptive behavior. This led to the inclusion of most mentally handicapped children within public education, and the functional significance of the educational classification system was greatly reduced. One version of this system is discussed in Hardman, Drew, and Egan (1996):

Educable	Tested IQ 55–70
Trainable	Tested IQ 40–55
Custodial	Tested IQ below 40

the intellectual honesty of the examiner—its intent is not to give an "easy out" in cases the present an assessment challenge. It is left to the examiner to determine when a given child or adolescent (or adult) cannot be validly assessed with quantitative instruments that have acceptable psychometric qualities.

Borderline Intellectual Functioning

Borderline Intellectual Functioning covers cases with tested intellectual ability in the range of 71 to 84. Borderline Intellectual Functioning may also be applied with IQ scores below 70 if there are no problems in adaptive behavior (First et al., 1995). It is worth reiterating that Borderline Intellectual Functioning is not a mental disorder in the language of DSM-IV. Instead, it is one of the categories in the chapter entitled "Other Conditions That May Be a Focus of Clinical Attention" (see the next Coding Note)—behavior problems and other complications that may justify clinical evaluation and treatment, but do not fall within the definition of Mental Disorders in DSM-IV. Borderline Intellectual Functioning is coded on Axis II; it is the only V

CODING NOTE   "V Codes"

In DSM-III and DSM-III-R the codes for all categories the section on Other Conditions That May Be a Focus of Clinical Attention began with the letter V. This is no longer completely the case in DSM-IV but the informal designation continues to be commonly used. A V code is a diagnosis but it is not a diagnosis of a Mental Disorder. It is a diagnosis of a condition which justifies professional response but does not meet the defining criteria for a Mental Disorder.

code to be included on this axis (see the Coding Note, Axes for Other Diagnoses, below). There is no functional impairment requirement for Borderline Intellectual Functioning, since this category is not a mental disorder. Nevertheless, the title of the chapter in which it appears suggests that the limited cognitive abilities have some deleterious consequences in the individual's life. The school psychologist will find that the V codes in general are both indispensably useful in assessing children and adolescents, and extremely frustrating in their lack of specificity and objectivity. Unfortunately, there are no criterion sets for the V codes to help encourage their consistent application.

Associated Problems and Diagnoses

Children with retarded intellectual functioning are at elevated risk for other behavior problems (Campbell & Malone, 1991; Einfeld & Aman, 1995). Greater than base rate prevalences for aggressive behavior, self-injurious behaviors, stereotypic behaviors, overactivity, and language problems are reported for children and adolescents diag-

CODING NOTE   Axes for Other Diagnoses

Learning Disorders, Communication Disorders, and Developmental Coordination Disorder are all coded on Axis I. This is a change from DSM-III-R where "Developmental Disorders" were coded on Axis II along with Mental Retardation. Only Mental Retardation, the V code Borderline Intellectual Functioning, and the Personality Disorders are on Axis II in DSM-IV.

nosed with MR (Aman, Hammer, & Rojahn, 1993; Bregman, 1991; Jacobson, 1982; Scott, 1994). A 6-year study by Menolascino and associates found "the entire range of psychiatric diagnoses" represented (Menolascino, 1988, p. 111), including a significant over-representation of Schizophrenia (DSM-III criteria). Instead of explaining these problems away as "part of the retardation," educators will serve young people with MR better by recognizing their associated mental health problems and treating these emotional and behavioral disturbances whenever possible. An examiner must realize that there is nothing about MR that protects a young person from other behavior problems, even if these are not differentially associated with MR. A negative change in a child's or adolescent's level of adjustment should lead to a high index of suspicion in the examiner regarding possible new difficulties, either environmental stresses or comorbid mental disorders. In my experience with developmentally disabled clients, I have seen both Major Depressive Episodes and Manic Episodes, that were missed in evaluations, despite obvious deteriorations in performance. The client's significant problems with depression and agitation were not recognized as potential indications of treatable disorders—sometimes with disastrous results.

In Mild to Moderate MR, the other diagnostic categories of DSM-IV have reasonable applicability, although even this statement is not as well supported with empirical data as would be desirable. With increasing severity of intellectual deficit, however, there is concern regarding the validity of categories developed primarily for individuals with normal intelligence (Einfeld & Aman, 1995). At the same time, the likelihood of associated behavior and emotional problems appears to increase with increasing severity of MR (Campbell & Malone, 1991; Einfeld & Aman, 1995). In my own work with retarded children and adolescents, I have often had occasion to use residual (Not Otherwise Specified or NOS) diagnoses. Einfeld and Aman (1995) suggest that multivariate analyses of behavioral and emotional symptoms in youth with MR yield some consistent dimensions of disturbance. Potentially relevant diagnoses from DSM-IV pertaining to these areas are shown in Table 8.1.

Several authors have discussed modifications of the DSM diagnostic criteria to increase their sensitivity and applicability to comorbid mental disorders in individuals with MR (King, DeAntonio, McCracken, Forness, & Ackerland, 1994; Reiss, 1994b; Szymanski, 1994). As with any modification of the DSM-IV diagnostic criteria, the examiner has the responsibility of being very clear and explicit about the basis on which a diagnosis is being made. Kay (1989) suggested that psychometric testing could be useful in making a differ-

TABLE 8.1. DSM-IV Diagnoses to Be Considered in Regard to Other Symptoms of Disturbance in Populations with MR

Area of disturbance	Diagnoses/conditions to be ruled in/out
Aggressive/antisocial behavior	Conduct Disorder Oppositional Defiant Disorder Disruptive Behavior Disorder NOS Adjustment Disorder With Disturbance of Conduct Adjustment Disorder With Mixed Disturbance of Emotions and Conduct Child or Adolescent Antisocial Behavior (not a Mental Disorder)
Social withdrawal	Social Phobia Anxiety Disorder NOS Adjustment Disorder, Unspecified Disorder of Infancy, Childhood, or Adolescence NOS
Self-injurious behavior	Stereotypic Movement Disorder
Hyperactivity	Attention-Deficit/Hyperactivity Disorder (ADHD) ADHD NOS
Inappropriate verbalizations	Disorder of Infancy, Childhood, or Adolescence NOS Personality Disorder NOS Unspecified Mental Disorder (nonpsychotic)

ential diagnosis between MR and psychosis, but I am not aware of replication of this work.

King et al. (1994) comment that many individuals with a diagnosis of MR do not fit neatly into a single diagnostic category. Comorbidity among different diagnoses is very common, as are subsyndromal presentations. A young person with MR may show features of a Mood or Anxiety Disorder that do not meet full criteria for a diagnosis, but do substantially interfere with his or her adjustment and complicate the case. Provisional and "rule-out" diagnoses are often found in the charts of retarded clients (King et al., 1994). As I have noted above, the use of the NOS classification opinion within the major DSM-IV diagnostic groupings has proved very helpful in my work with children and adolescents with MR who show other behavioral problems.

A few disorders that commonly co-occur with MR are worth mentioning specifically here. Stereotypic movements (motor behaviors that are repetitive, nonfunctional, and self-stimulatory) are often seen in association with MR, especially as the severity of MR increases (Campbell & Malone, 1991); if such behaviors become troublesome enough to justify a treatment focus the diagnosis of Stereotypic Movement Disorder (discussed in Chapter 7) can be made concurrently with that of MR. The specifier With Self-Injurious Behavior is noted if applicable. Self-injurious behavior is associated both with the severity of MR and with environmental influences (Campbell & Malone, 1991).

A diagnosis of MR can be made concurrently with a diagnosis of a Pervasive Developmental Disorder (PDD), and in fact these are commonly comorbid conditions (see Chapter 9). DSM-IV suggests that 75–80% of clients with PDD also show MR (p. 45). A child who shows MR, Autistic Disorder (or another PDD), and repetitive self-injurious behavior should not receive an additional diagnosis of Stereotypic Movement Disorder. A diagnosis of a PDD precludes a concurrent diagnosis of Stereotypic Movement Disorder.

If the MR is caused after a period of normal mental development and functioning, the additional diagnosis of Dementia (discussed in more detail later in this chapter) is justified. Considering pragmatic issues in determining premorbid level of functioning, DSM-IV suggests that the diagnosis of Dementia not be used prior to the ages of 4–6. The text further suggests that a concurrent diagnosis of Dementia with MR only be used for those cases where the essential features of the clinical situation are not adequately captured by the solitary diagnosis of MR.

LEARNING DISORDERS AND RELATED PROBLEMS

Definition and Classification of Learning Disorders

Consistent with most discussions of learning problems, DSM-IV defines a Learning Disorder as existing "when the individual's achievement on individually administered, standardized tests in reading, mathematics, or written expression is substantially below that expected for age, schooling, and level of intelligence" (p. 46). This is one of the few categories where psychological testing is explicitly considered, and there is discussion of "substantially below" as reflecting a discrepancy of two standard deviations or more between measures of academic achievement and ability (tested intelligence). There remain, however, many unresolved issues in how to operationalize the concept of a Learning Disorder. This is the central conflict in efforts to delineate the boundaries of learning problems. Poor school performance can arise from a multitude of influences. A Mental Disorder per se is neither necessary nor sufficient to explain school failure. In addition to this enduring puzzle, ongoing research continues to challenge traditional ideas about learning problems (see, e.g., Shaywitz, Escobar, Shaywitz, Fletcher, & Makuch, 1990; Shaywitz, Shaywitz, Fletcher, & Escobar, 1990).

DSM-IV has relaxed most of the exclusion rules for Learning Disorders. In contrast to previous editions, DSM-IV permits these disorders to be diagnosed concurrently with conditions of sensory, motor, neurological, and intellectual impairment, but only if the discrepancy between a child's academic skill performance and general intellectual level is significant and cannot be adequately explained by the other specific deficits or limitations. The practical applications of concurrent diagnoses of MR and a Learning Disorder are limited; only special cases (e.g., Mild MR and a very severe and focused Learning Disorder) are likely to qualify. The conceptual implications are, however, significant. The Learning Disorder diagnoses in DSM-IV are written in a much more flexible manner than in previous editions, with a corresponding increase in the examiner's responsibility to assess each individual case carefully.

The classification of Learning Disorders in DSM-IV reflects the primary academic areas of difficulty. Three specific categories and a residual diagnosis are provided: Reading Disorder, Mathematics Disorder, Disorder of Written Expression, and Learning Disorder NOS. (Because the three specific Learning Disorders are so often comorbid with one another, I discuss them individually in more detail under "Associated Problems and Diagnoses," below.) For a solid background in the complexities of attempting to subdivide learning problems in meaningful and useful ways the reader is referred to Hooper and Willis (1989). The next IDEA Note sets forth how Learning Disorders relate to eligibility for services under IDEA.

Learning Disorder Not Otherwise Specified

In my clinical work, the DSM-IV diagnosis of Learning Disorder NOS is invaluable. This category can be used to cover presentations of learning problems that do not meet the specific requirements of the three identified patterns but do cause significant problems for academic success and/or personal distress for the young people involved (i.e., problems that constitute mental disorders). At the same time, it is imperative that the examiner exercise due professional integrity and

IDEA NOTE   Learning Disorders and IDEA

"Specific learning disabilities" are identified qualifying conditions for special services under IDEA. A Learning Disorder identified in DSM-IV will establish a "specific learning disability" and thus qualify a child for services under IDEA. Differences between the DSM-IV and IDEA views of learning handicaps may arise, however, out of particular state or district formulations of specific learning disabilities, which often specify a magnitude of discrepancy between measures of aptitude and achievement required to qualify a child for services (e.g., 22 standard score points). As I have noted in my text discussion, DSM-IV requires achievement that is "substantially below that expected for age, schooling, and level of intelligence" (p. 46). An exact operational definition of "substantially below" is not given; DSM-IV indicates that substantially below "is usually defined as a discrepancy of more than two standard deviations between achievement and IQ" (p. 46), but goes on to state that smaller discrepancies (between one and two standard deviations) may be used if an individual's tested intelligence has been compromised by a cognitive processing disorder, a comorbid mental disorder, a general medical condition, or ethnic or cultural background factors. As is always the case in DSM-IV, the professional judgment of the examiner is the ultimate deciding factor. Although it is clear that educational classifications are not always decided by a strict adherence to state or district formulations (MacMillan, et al., 1996), a critical difference is that in DSM-IV the decisive role of clinical judgment is seen as justified and desirable (p. xxiii). In short, IDEA's concept of a "specific learning disability" is essentially the same as DSM-IV's concept of A Learning Disorder, but the boundaries of classification do not always perfectly coincide between the two systems.

---

personal honesty. Learning Disorder NOS should reflect the basic concept of a Learning Disorder; that is, it should involve academic difficulty and failure that cannot be better accounted for by a low level of general intellectual functioning, inadequate effort, low subcultural valuation of school achievement, or the expected disruption of life caused by many mental disorders (especially Disruptive Behavior Disorders, Mood Disorders, Anxiety Disorders, and Psychotic Disorders). There is a real danger that the more socially acceptable diagnostic classification of Learning Disorder NOS will be used when other conceptualizations (Mild MR, Borderline Intellectual Functioning, or Academic Problem—the latter two, of course are not mental disorders) may be more valid. I can only suggest that we are all ultimately best served when diagnostic classification systems (including DSM-IV) are used as honestly and accurately as possible.

A particular application of Learning Disorder NOS that will be of interest to some school psychologists is the designation of those learning problems identified as "nonverbal." The topic of nonverbal learning disabilities has received a great deal of recent interest because of the research and publications of Byron Rourke (Rourke, 1987, 1988, 1989; Rourke, Del Dotto, Rourke, & Casey, 1990), but the concept is not a new one. Myklebust (1975) presented one early discussion of this topic. Associations between primary difficulties with visual–spatial relationships, constructional performances, part–whole processing, and other cognitive and behavioral phenomena are topics of current interest (Semrud-Klikeman & Hynd, 1990). Within the framework of DSM-IV, a nonverbal learning disability is coded as Learning Disorder NOS. When an examiner is using this category, it is appropriate and valuable to identify as clearly as possible the specific deficits in the child's ability structure. Nonverbal learning problems may be associated with other mental disorders, including Developmental Coordination Disorder (Henderson, Barnett, & Henderson, 1994), Asperger's Disorder (Klin, Volkmar, Sparrow, Cicchetti, & Rourke, 1995), and other emotional and personality problems (Hellgren, Gillberg, Bagenholm, & Gillberg, 1994).

Academic Problem

Academic Problem, like Borderline Intellectual Functioning, is a V code. This classification can be used to cover cases of academic problems that are not attributable to a mental disorder. The text gives the example of a young person's failing classes in the absence of a Learning or Communication Disorder or any other mental disorder that would account for these effects. In my experience, the designation of Academic Problem should serve as a cue for further investigation into a child's or adolescent's adjustment, family circumstances, social relationships, and environment. Either abrupt or gradual changes in school performance may be early objective signs of difficulty with the many developmental hurdles of childhood and adolescence (peer pressures, sexuality, substance use experimentation, lifestyle choices, or the demands of part-time employment on time and energy). Poor school performance is one of the best-established risk factors for dropping out of school (Oakland, 1992), and it deserves serious evaluation and aggressive assistance.

Associated Problems and Diagnoses

The linkages between learning problems and other cognitive, behavioral, and emotional characteristics of children are complex and not fully understood—a reality well appreciated by practicing school psychologists. Statistical associations have been reported between Learning Disorders in particular and academic underachievement in general, as well as between Learning Disorders and a number of other major mental disorders: Conduct Disorder, Oppositional Defiant Disorder, ADHD, Major Depressive Disorder, Dysthymic Disorder, and Anxiety Disorders. A history of Developmental Coordination Disorder (see below) and/or Communication Disorders may be found in the background of many children with Learning Disorders; these previous difficulties may have largely resolved or may never have been serious enough actually to warrant diagnosis. Finally, the specific Learning Disorders defined in DSM-IV are often comorbid in a given child, and multiple diagnoses are probably the rule rather than the exception.

A good deal of attention has been paid recently to the social problems of children with learning disabilities. These may be a significant factor in the morbidity associated with Learning Disorders, especially for the difficulties labeled "nonverbal learning disabilities." The social learning problems of children with Learning Disorders may be one important influence contributing to an elevated risk for personality trait disturbance and Personality Disorders in adults with a childhood history of learning problems (Khan, Cowan, & Roy, 1997). However, as is true of many other topics regarding Learning Disorders, much additional research is needed to clarify these questions. I am convinced that advances in the empirical and conceptual understanding of Learning Disorders will require the development of more specific categories and subcategories of this heterogeneous diagnostic grouping.

Comorbidities with and among the Specific Learning Disorders

Reading problems are among the most common academic difficulties encountered in school settings and are certainly the most often investigated. No distinction is made in DSM-IV between Reading Disorder involving more phonological processing errors and that involving more visual–spatial processing difficulty (e.g., "dysphonetic dyslexia" vs. "dyseidetic dyslexia"). There are strong associations between Reading Disorder and problems with phonological processing, and a history (not necessarily current) of Phonological Disorder may be found. Frequent comorbid associations with the other two specific Learning Disorder categories are noted. Reading Disorder also shows associations with other mental disorders, especially ADHD, Disruptive Behavior Disorders, and (in older children or adolescents) Mood Disorders and Substance Use Disorders. Untangling the nature, direction, and causality of these associations is an ongoing task and may be complicated by gender-specific pathways (Frick et al., 1991; Smart, Sanson, & Prior, 1966; Shaywitz, Shaywitz, et al., 1990).

Mathematics Disorder and Disorder of Written Expression are provided in DSM-IV as additional diagnoses of specific learning problems. Other than title and axis changes, little has altered in the presentation of all three specific Learning Disorder categories from DSM-III-R. The diagnoses were called Developmental Reading Disorder, Developmental Arithmetic Disorder, and Developmental Expressive Writing Disorder previously and were coded on Axis II, along with the Specific and Pervasive Developmental Disorders and MR. Only MR, Personality Disorders, and the V code Borderline Intellectual Functioning are coded on Axis II in DSM-IV (see the Coding Note, Axes for Other Diagnoses, on p. 131). Although clinical experience suggests that learning disability confined to arithmetic skills does occur among children and adolescents, the unique occurrence of writing problems is less clearly established. Problems of written expression usually occur in association with reading problems. A given child may actually meet criteria for all three of the specific DSM-IV Learning Disorder diagnoses.

The text of DSM-IV acknowledges that less is known about Disorder of Written Expression than about the other Learning Disorders, and that the available assessment tools are less satisfactory. The diagnostic criteria allow for "functional assessments of writing skills" as an alternative to standardized tests for establishment of Disorder of Written Expression; this formal exception is not provided for with the other two diagnoses. One fine point is worth noting: Spelling errors alone or poor handwriting alone is not usually diagnosed as Disorder of Written Expression (p. 52). Poor spelling usually occurs in the context of Reading Disorder, except for the interesting and unusual cases of isolated spelling disability with good reading skills (so-called "benign spelling dyspraxia"). Poor handwriting may be a symptom of Developmental Coordination Disorder (see below). The boundaries between these various categories are conceptually problematic, and diagnosis of the individual child will ultimately require the examiner's best judgment as to the diagnosis or combination of diagnoses that most meaningfully and fully captures the essential features of a particular young person's difficulties.

Developmental Coordination Disorder

Developmental Coordination Disorder is the only member of the "Motor Skills Disorder" section in the "Disorders Usually First Diagnosed in Infancy, Childhood, or Adolescence" chapter; it is identified as an impairment in the development of motor coordination interferes significantly with scholastic achievement or general daily activities. The disorder category is not due to a general medical condition and this diagnosis is not made concurrently with that of a PDD. It can be made together with a diagnosis of MR, but the degree of motor incoordination must be greater than that which would be expected as an associated feature of the MR. This disorder can also be diagnosed concurrently with ADHD. It is discussed here, however, because of its particularly close association with the Learning Disorders. The next IDEA Note sets forth how this disorder relates to eligibility for services under IDEA.

Developmental Coordination Disorder was introduced in DSM-III-R to facilitate research into the possible links between various aspects of development and learning and behavior problems. Nonspecific motor incoordination has been treated by some clinicians as a "soft" or "minor" neurological sign. There is little empirical literature on this DSM diagnosis, and it is probably too soon to know how useful it will prove. Related concepts, however, have been studied and found to be associated with academic difficulties. Fletcher-Flinn, Elmes, and Strugnell (1997) reported on a group of 30 children in New Zealand diagnosed with "congenital developmental coordination disorder" and found that 25% had severe reading difficulties and 30% severe spelling disabilities. The spelling problems were associ-

---

IDEA NOTE   Developmental Coordination Disorder and IDEA

Although I know of no relevant cases, it seems to me that a DSM-IV diagnosis of Developmental Coordination Disorder can form the basis for a qualification of a child as eligible for special services under IDEA through the "other health impaired" category, if the disorder adversely affects the child's educational performance. The functional impairment criterion for the category will have special significance if this diagnosis is being used to qualify inclusion under IDEA: "The disturbance in Criterion A significantly interferes with academic achievement or activities of daily living" (p. 55).

---

ated with visual discrimination, but the reading difficulties were not; phonological awareness and spelling problems were associated with reading difficulties. Associations between motor control and clumsiness, visual–spatial perception, and attention problems continue to be investigated (Hellgren et al., 1994; Henderson et al., 1994).

I have found the phenomenon indexed by the diagnosis of Developmental Coordination Disorder in several children and adolescents with learning problems, especially those who fit the so-called "nonverbal learning disability" pattern. I would suggest careful evaluation of Developmental Coordination Disorder as a possible comorbid diagnosis in children diagnosed with Mathematics Disorder, which has also been linked by Rourke to his concept of nonverbal learning disabilities. Increased awareness of this category should lead to a better understanding of the links among sensory, motor, cognitive, and academic development in children.

COMMUNICATION DISORDERS

Also included in the "Disorders Usually First Diagnosed in Infancy, Childhood, or Adolescence" chapter are the Communication Disorders. This section covers several language and speech problems often found in youth: Expressive Language Disorder, Mixed Expressive–Receptive Language Disorder, Phonological Disorder, Stuttering, and Communication Disorder NOS. These diagnoses are all coded on Axis I (see the Coding Note, Axes for Other Diagnoses, on p. 131). Although written in response to DSM-III, a good introduction to this specialty area for the school and child clinical psychologist remains Cantwell and Baker's 1987 text. The next IDEA Note sets forth how the Communication Disorders relate to eligibility for services under IDEA.

IDEA NOTE   Communication Disorders and IDEA

Speech or language impairments are identified qualifying conditions for special services under IDEA. Communication Disorders as defined by DSM-IV typically equate with speech or language handicaps as identified by IDEA, although it is possible that a particular state or school district may formulate very specific operational definitions of a speech or language impairment that are more restrictive than the criteria in DSM-IV (cf. the IDEA Note on p. 136).

Communication Disorders may be associated with the Learning Disorders and with cognitive problems. The linkage between reading problems and an earlier history of articulation or language problems has been discussed above. Communication Disorders can also be a sequelae of traumatic brain injury (TBI) in children (Ewing-Cobbs, Levin, Eisenberg, & Fletcher, 1987; Jordan, Ozanne, & Murdoch, 1990; Jordan, Murdoch, Buttsworth, & Hudson-Tennent, 1995). In children, a transient "acquired aphasia" may be associated with a general medical condition such as encephalitis or TBI. If the language disruption persists beyond the acute recovery period for the general medical condition, then a diagnosis of a Communication Disorder become appropriate (p. 57). Communication Disorders secondary to TBI may persist over extended periods and have important implications for academic and social adjustment. A younger age at the time of injury and greater severity of injury are both associated with poorer outcome (Ewing-Cobbs, Miner, Fletcher, & Levin, 1989; Jordan, Ozanne, & Murdoch, 1988; Yorkston, Jaffe, Polissar, Liao, & Fay, 1997). Communication Disorders secondary to TBI may involve both oral and written language production (Yorkston et al., 1997), and an associated diagnosis of Disorder of Written Expression may be warranted. (TBI is discussed further under "Cognitive Problems," below.)

Two primary language disorders are presented: Expressive Language Disorder and Mixed Receptive–Expressive Language Disorder. (The next Coding Note describes recent changes in the ICD-9-CM

CODING NOTE   Coding Changes for Communication Disorders

As mentioned earlier in this book (see the Coding Note on p. 49), the ICD-9-CM is annually reviewed and updated by a federal committee. Following the submission and review process described in that same Coding Note the final coding changes are published as an Interim Final Notice in the May–June issue of the *Federal Register*. Two recent publications by the American Psychiatric Association (1996a, 1996b) present 23 updated codes affecting DSM-IV diagnostic categories and 7 updated codes from DSM-IV Appendix G. One of the categories affected is Mixed Receptive-Expressive Language Disorder. This category previously had the same ICD-9-CM code as Expressive Language Disorder; both were coded 315.31. The revised coding differentiates between these two patterns. Expressive Language Disorder remains the same, and Mixed Receptive–Expressive Language Disorder is now coded as 315.32.

---

coding of these two disorders.) Neither of these is diagnosed concurrently with a PDD. Either can be diagnosed concurrently with MR (as well as sensory or motor conditions) if the language deficit is in excess of what could be reasonably expected on the basis of the MR alone. Receptive language difficulty (problems of oral comprehension) preclude the diagnosis of Expressive Language Disorder. Receptive language disturbance is almost inevitably associated with problems of oral expression; hence the use of the title Mixed Receptive–Expressive Language Disorder in place of the more common label "receptive language disorder."

Two primary speech disorders are presented: Phonological Disorder (called Developmental Articulation Disorder in DSM-III-R) and Stuttering. The definitions of both are typical of discussions within the field of speech pathology. Speech problems may be diagnosed concurrently with MR or with neurological disorders involving sensory or speech–motor deficit if the speech disturbance is greater than could be reasonably accounted for by the comorbid condition. Phonological Disorder will be of interest to many school psychologists, because a history of articulation difficulties is common in some cases of Reading Disorder (as noted earlier) and may help identify a phonological processing pattern of reading disability. Articulation problems, which often improve or resolve with age, are associated with a variety of concurrent developmental problems (Coplan & Gleason, 1988). Improved norms for assessing clarity of speech in preschool children (Coplan & Gleason, 1988) should facilitate continuing research into the linkages between speech, language, cognitive, and behavioral development.

The category of Communication Disorder NOS covers language and speech disorders identified by specialists in this field that are not formally classified by DSM-IV—voice disorders, developmental dysarthrias, primary developmental anomia, and other phenomena of primary concern to speech and language pathologists. Although these problems merge into areas in which psychologists have limited training or expertise, some familiarity with allied health fields will enhance school psychologists' ability to interact with other professionals who play either established or developing roles within schools (Leeper, 1992; Paul, 1995).

Finally, it may be worth mentioning Selective Mutism (discussed in Chapter 7) briefly here, because it is sometimes thought of as a communication problem. However, DSM-IV does not group it with the Communication Disorders (it is placed in the "Other Disorders of Infancy, Childhood, or Adolescence" section). Moreover, as noted in Chapter 7, Selective Mutism is probably best conceptualized as an anxiety problem (Dummit et al., 1997). Only about one-third of children with Selective Mutism have a history of other speech or language problems (Steinhausen & Juzi, 1996).

COGNITIVE PROBLEMS

The "Delirium, Dementia, and Amnestic and Other Cognitive Disorders" chapter of DSM-IV covers clinically significant deficits in mental ability that represent a change from a previous level of functioning. These disorders were referred to as Organic Mental Disorders in DSM-III-R; this label was dropped because of concern that it implied an absence of biological basis for "nonorganic" mental disorders. Strub and Black (1988) suggested the designation "neurobehavioral disorders" for these biologically based problems of mental processing, but the authors of DSM-IV opted out of advancing a summary label. These categories have their most common applications with adults, but because several possible applications pertain to children and adolescents, the school psychologist should have some knowledge of this group of diagnoses.

Delirium

Delirium involves acute disturbances in consciousness and cognition. Strub and Black (1988) label these disorders "acute confusional states," which conveys a clear picture of the problem, but the more traditional term remains popular and is used in DSM-IV. Delirium in children and adolescents presents in the context of serious medical conditions that bring the youth into a health care setting.

Dementia

Dementia involves a loss of previously established mental ability. In DSM-IV, a Dementia is defined by a demonstrable impairment in memory plus one (or more) other disturbances of mental ability (aphasia, apraxia, agnosia, or deficit in executive functioning). The reader should be aware that not all conceptualizations of dementia require a memory deficit as one of the defining features (Strub & Black, 1988). Also, in contrast to some usages of "dementia" that imply a progressive and nonreversible course, in DSM-IV Dementia identifies a pattern of cognitive deficits without assumption about the course or stability of these impairments. The disorders in the "Dementia" section of DSM-IV are further classified by etiology. Of special interest to the school psychologist will be Dementia Due to Head Trauma, an unacceptably frequent occurrence in school-age individuals. Dementia due to Other General Medical Conditions (e.g., lead encephalopathy) is also seen in school settings. In addition, it may be useful for the school psychologist to be aware of associations between Dementia and other medical disorders of relevance to educators. For instance, it appears that all individuals with trisomy 21 (Down's syndrome), a common etiology of MR, will develop the neurological characteristics of Alzheimer's disease in their adult lives (Pietrini et al., 1997). It has not been completely established that they will manifest Dementia of the Alzheimer's Type (DAT) as defined in DSM-IV. As an interesting contrast, it also appears that individuals with MR secondary to trisomy 21 may not show the association between MR and other comorbid MD usually demonstrated with MR (Campbell & Malone, 1991).

It is worth noting briefly that the diagnosis of DAT in DSM-IV does not necessarily imply that the dementia has definitely determined to be due to Alzheimer's disease (a specific neuropathology). At this time Alzheimer's disease can only be conclusively established on the basis of neurological tissue analysis (e.g., a biopsy or autopsy of brain tissue). The DSM-IV diagnosis of DAT is based on a behavioral pattern of cognitive deficits; many of these cases with be found upon autopsy not to have had Alzheimer's disease, but vascular dementia, Pick's disease, or some other neuropathology or combination of neuropathologies. The text of DSM-IV is somewhat inconsistent—acknowledging that DAT is a behavioral diagnosis made on the basis of exclusion (pp. 139–140), but then suggesting that a concurrent diagnosis of Alzheimer's disease should be coded on Axis III. In fact, many diagnoses of DAT currently made under DSM-IV would probably be more properly made as Dementia NOS.

If an individual has only a problem in memory, without another area of cognitive deficit, the diagnosis should be an Amnestic Disorder. One will occasionally see Amnestic Disorder Due to Head Trauma in adolescents or children. Like Dementia, Amnestic Disorders in DSM-IV can be temporary or persistent.

Cognitive Disorder Not Otherwise Specified

Cognitive Disorder NOS is the residual classification for acquired deficits in cognitive ability that do not meet the essential features for the three identified patterns (Delirium, Dementia, Amnestic Disorders). One important application is the identification of a possible "postconcussional disorder." The concept of an identifiable pattern of mental difficulty and neurobehavioral symptoms following so-called "mild head injury" (i.e., head injury without definitive neurological signs) has been investigated and discussed for several decades in the neurological and neuropsychological literature. In Appendix B, "Criteria Sets and Axes Provided for Further Study," DSM-IV gives a set of research criteria for the proposed "postconcussional Disorder." In cases where this criterion set is applied, the formal diagnosis should be coded as Cognitive Disorder NOS.

Problems Related to Traumatic Brain Injury

The topic of TBI (discussed above in regard to Communication Disorders) has received increasing interest within school settings since the acceptance of TBI as a qualifying condition for special education services. The next IDEA Note sets forth how TBI relates to eligibility for services under IDEA. Acute brain injuries account for approximately 100,000 pediatric hospital admissions each year in the United States; about 93% of these are classified as mild (Kraus, Fife, & Conroy, 1987). Each year approximately 29,000 youth between the ages of 0 and 19 acquire some degree of residual disability secondary to TBI

IDEA NOTE   TBI and IDEA

When P.L. 94-142 was revised as IDEA (P.L. 101-476) in 1990, the category of TBI was added as an identified qualifying condition establishing eligibility for special education and other services through the school system. TBI is *not* a mental disorder in the DSM-IV classification system, although it may be an etiological factor in several different disorders. TBI should be indicated as a general medical condition on Axis III. Deterioration or loss in a child's or adolescent's mental functioning and/or behavioral adjustment caused by TBI is a mental disorder and should be coded on Axis I according to the pattern of symptoms: Dementia Due to Head Trauma, Amnestic Disorder Due to Head Trauma, Cognitive Disorder NOS, Personality Change Due to Head Injury, Psychotic Disorder Due Head Trauma, Mood Disorder Due to Head Trauma, or Anxiety Disorder Due to Head Trauma. When associated with TBI, any of these would presumably qualify a child for services under IDEA. Note that a Personality Change Due to a General Medical Condition (such as TBI) is the only occasion in which a "personality diagnosis" is made on Axis I. Personality Disorders (when a general medical condition is not established as the cause) are classified on Axis II.

(Kraus, Rock, & Hemyari, 1990). Finally, almost all children who survive the initial trauma leading to TBI will eventually return to school (Carney & Schoenbrodt, 1994).

TBI in children is a risk factor for cognitive and behavior problems (Begali, 1992; Rutter, 1981). Although the association between severe TBI and behavioral and adaptive problems is well established (Brown, Chadwick, Shaffer, Rutter, & Traub, 1981; Fay et al., 1994; Fletcher, Ewing-Cobbs, Miner, Levin, & Eisenberg, 1990; Knights, Ivan, Ventureyra, et al., 1991; Max, Smith, et al., 1997; Rivara, Jaffe, Fay, et al., 1993), the relation between mild TBI and psychiatric outcome has been more widely debated (Max & Dunisch, 1997). Development of a "novel" psychiatric disorder (i.e., a disorder unobserved prior to injury) during the first 3 months following TBI in children and adolescents is associated with greater severity of the injury, lower preinjury intellectual ability, a premorbid history of behavior problems, and a family history of psychiatric problems (Max, Smith, et al., 1997). Common initial cognitive difficulties following TBI include problems with general intellectual functioning, cognitive flexibility, memory, and verbal fluency (Slater & Bassett, 1988), which can have serious implications for a child's or adolescent's return to school and community. Careful assessment and follow-up by the school psychologist can greatly facilitate such a young person's successful reentry into their academic and social worlds. Awareness and communication of common associated symptoms of TBI can help minimize adjustment problems. Greater vulnerability to fatigue, illness, chemical influences (prescription, over-the-counter, and illicit drugs), and stress are typical sequelae of TBI; all can have significant educational implications. The longitudinal studies of Max and his colleagues (Max, Robin, et al., 1997) found that injury severity, preinjury family functioning, and preinjury adjustment history were all related to the continued presence of "novel" psychiatric problems during the second year following TBI.

Although it is desirable for the school psychologist to be sensitive to the multiple potential consequences of TBI in children, it is also necessary to recognize that a history of recent TBI does not automatically mean that neurological insult is the causal agent in any adjustment problems. There is no unique pattern of maladjustment associated with in children; the problems seen are essentially the same as those of a general group of children with mental health difficulties (Max, Sharma, & Qurashi, 1997). Chronic problems that predate the head injury are obviously not caused by TBI. The most appropriate interpretation of exacerbations of long-standing adjustment difficulties following TBI is very challenging and should usually be made cautiously.

CHAPTER 9

♦♦♦

Highly Atypical Symptom Patterns: Pervasive Developmental Disorders and Psychoses

♦

OVERVIEW

The conceptualization of the most severe behavioral disorders in DSM-IV reflects the interaction of two considerations: (1) the appearance of qualitatively distinctive and very disruptive signs and symptoms (e.g., psychotic symptoms, significant behavior deficits, stereotyped self-stimulation); and (2) temporal features of the disturbance (age of onset, duration). The Pervasive Developmental Disorders (PDDs) involve major disruptions in various aspects of normal development—reciprocal social responsiveness, communication, an increasingly complex behavioral repertoire—as well as an onset early in life, either with or without a preceding period of normal development. The Psychotic Disorders involve characteristic symptoms (delusions, hallucinations, profound disorganization of behavior, negative symptoms) occurring over various periods of time (less than a month, 1–6 months, more than 6 months). These two groupings (plus a few other disorders in which psychotic symptoms may appear) represent the most recent attempts to define some of the most severe and puzzling disturbances of behavior and adjustment seen in human beings. Research continues, and it is doubtful that DSM-IV will represent the last word on marking the boundaries of the PDDs and the Psychotic Disorders; nevertheless, the formulations of DSM-IV appear to constitute both an advance over previous editions of DSM and a basis for reasonably objective and reliable evaluation.

PERVASIVE DEVELOPMENTAL DISORDERS

The occurrence of severe disorders in childhood associated not only with the behavioral deficits evident in Mental Retardation, but also with highly unusual behavioral excesses or "deviant" behavior, has been recognized for some time. Labels such as "childhood psychosis" and "childhood schizophrenia" were formally applied to such children, often in such an all-inclusive and noncritical manner that little meaning was conveyed (see, e.g., Creak, 1961, 1963). The current definition of these disorders as PDDs both highlights their essential features (multiple impairment in major areas of development and onset early in life) and helps differentiate these psychopathologies from the common forms of psychosis disorder seen in adolescents and adults. An important improvement in DSM-IV, from the perspective of both clinicians and researchers, is the increased differentiation of this group. By contrast with the two categories available in DSM-III-R (Autistic Disorder and PDD Not Otherwise Specified [NOS]), DSM-IV provides five PDDs that effectively capture many of the variations seen in child practice. The next Coding Note describes the changes in the multiaxial classification of the PDDs from DSM-III to DSM-IV, and the next IDEA Note sets forth how the PDDs relate to eligibility for services under IDEA.

Autistic Disorder

The most thoroughly investigated of the PDDs is autism. The Autistic Disorder of DSM-IV represents a return to the relatively specific Infantile Autism diagnosis of DSM-III and identifies a population similar to that covered by the original "Kanner's syndrome," in contrast to the more sensitive and less specific criterion set of DSM-III-R. This is welcomed by most researchers in this area, some of whom continued using the DSM-III criterion set despite the appearance of DSM-III-R. The effect of the changes in DSM-IV is to reduce the population of children identified as showing Autistic Disorder to a more homogeneous group of children with multiple and severe problems in social responsiveness, language development, and elaboration of goal-directed behavior.

Additional Diagnoses to Be Considered

Mental Retardation occurs in up to 75–80% of children afflicted with Autistic Disorder and carries important prognostic significance. If a child's general intellectual functioning is compromised to a signifi-

CODING NOTE   The Multiaxial Classification of PDDs
from DSM-III to DSM-IV

In DSM-III, the PDDs (with the primary diagnosis of Infantile Autism) were coded on Axis I. Only the Specific Developmental Disorders (learning, language, and some speech disorders) and Personality Disorders were coded on Axis II.

In DSM-III-R, the PDDs (with the primary diagnosis of Autistic Disorder) were moved to Axis II, along with Mental Retardation and the V code Borderline Intellectual Functioning. The Specific Developmental Disorders (now including the subgroups of Academic Skills disorders, Language and Speech Disorders, and Motor Skill Disorder) and Personality Disorders remained on Axis II.

In DSM-IV, the PDDs—now with four primary diagnoses (including Autistic Disorder) and an NOS category—have been returned to Axis I, along with the Learning Disorders, Motor Skills Disorder, and Communication Disorders. Mental Retardation, Borderline Intellectual Functioning, and Personality Disorders remain on Axis II. Only the Personality Disorders have consistently remained on Axis II across the three presentations of DSM as a multiaxial diagnostic system.

cant degree (IQ less than 70), the additional diagnosis of Mental Retardation is made. Neurological problems associated with Autistic Disorder include seizure disorders, which usually develop in adolescence. There is an association between Mental Retardation and seizure disorder development in children with Autistic Disorder, and both are associated with a poorer prognosis (Morgan, 1990).

Precluded Diagnoses

Stereotyped, nonpurposeful motor movements (self-stimulation) are also characteristic of children with Autistic Disorder. The work of Lovaas suggests that these responses are not benign; especially at very high frequencies, they actively compete against most appropriate learning. But because they are an associated symptom, a concurrent diagnosis of Stereotypic Movement Disorder should not be made. Various (e.g., Developmental Coordination Disorder, the Communication Disorders, Pica, Rumination Disorder, Selective Mutism, Reactive Attachment Disorder) are also precluded under the general hierarchical arrangement of DSM categories, in which more pervasive categories subsume more specific diagnoses (in most cases).

IDEA NOTE   PDD and IDEA

For the purposes of IDEA, "autism" has been defined as follows:

Autism means a developmental disability significantly affecting verbal and nonverbal communication and social interaction, generally evident before age 3, that adversely affects educational performance. Characteristics of autism include—irregularities and impairments in communication, engagement in repetitive activities and stereotyped movements, resistance to environmental change or change in daily routines, and unusual responses to sensory experiences. (U.S. Department of Education, 1991, p. 41271)

I believe that all children who receive a DSM-IV diagnosis of Autistic Disorder clearly fall within this qualifying classification. It is less clear whether the other DSM-IV PDDs (Rett's Disorder, Childhood Disintegrative Disorder [CDD], Asperger's Disorder, and PDD NOS) can be treated as "autism" for the purposes of IDEA. Rett's Disorder and CDD conceivably can be; PDD NOS may depending on the specific problems; and Asperger's Disorder probably cannot be, given the usually adequate communication associated with this syndrome. All of these other PDDs can, however, qualify relatively easily for services under IDEA because of the severity of functional impairment seen in children afflicted with these global disturbances of adjustment. Either the "seriously emotionally disturbed" category of Part B or the "other health impaired" category can be used to document the handicaps for academic, social, and personal adjustment associated with these PDDs.

Rett's Disorder

Rett's Disorder is a new category in DSM-IV. It is distinguished from other PDD by several of its symptoms (physical: deceleration of head growth; behavioral: development of stereotyped hand movements, development of poorly coordinated gait or trunk movement), its age of onset (intermediate between those of Autistic Disorder and Childhood Disintegrative Disorder [CDD]), and its sex ratio (all known cases are female). This is a very infrequent pattern (even relative to Autistic Disorder) and is unlikely to be seen in the typical school setting. Harris, Glasberg, and Ricca (1996) provide a nice discussion of symptom that help differentiate among Autistic Disorder, Rett's Disorder, and CDD. Girls with Rett's Disorder often show intense eye contact, teeth grinding, hyperventilation, and breath holding—

behaviors that are not typical of Autistic Disorder. The regression that characterizes Rett's Disorder also typically occurs developmentally sooner than that seen in CDD; children with CDD usually manifest a more sustained period of typical functioning.

Mental Retardation is common in children with Rett's Disorder and should be made as an additional diagnosis if present.

Childhood Disintegrative Disorder

CDD is another new diagnosis in DSM-IV, although the concept of a severe, regressive form of PDD has been discussed in the literature for some time (Volkmar & Rutter, 1995). The defining feature of CDD is a severe loss of previously acquired skills in communication, social relationships, and adaptive behavior and play, following at least 2 years of unremarkable growth and learning. Similar patterns previously described in the literature have been called "Heller's syndrome," "dementia infantilis," "disintegrative psychosis," or "disintegrative disorder." Although there is an empirical literature supporting CD as a real pattern (Volkmar & Rutter, 1995), it is a rare disorder (even relative to Autistic Disorder) and is not commonly seen in general school psychology practice. As noted above, the review by Harris et al. (1996) facilitates discrimination among CDD, Rett's Disorder, and Autistic Disorder. Volkmar, Klin, Marans, and McDougle (1996) provide a helpful tabular comparison of autism, Asperger's Disorder, Rett's Disorder, CDD, and PDD NOS.

Mental Retardation is common in children with CDD and should be made as an additional diagnosis if present.

Asperger's Disorder

Asperger's Disorder as identified by DSM-IV includes the impairment in social responsiveness and constricted repertoire of goal-directed activity seen in Autistic Disorder, but is characterized by normal language development and does not include deficiencies in cognitive development, self-help skills, or nonsocial adaptive behavior. One positive effect of the addition of this category to DSM-IV is that it will certainly spur research on this and related "autistic-like" phenomena and lead to a better empirical data base. Asperger's Disorder has been conceived of by some as a mild form of Autistic Disorder and by others as a separate and unique problem (Volkmar, Klin, Schultz, et al., 1996). Although few formal data are available, it appears reasonable to assume that the school psychologist is much more likely to encounter children with Asperger's Disorder in public school settings than children with Autistic Disorder.

Mental Retardation is not typical of children with Asperger's Disorder, but learning problems are. The diagnostic boundaries between Asperger's Disorder and high-functioning individuals with Autistic Disorder on the one hand, and Asperger's Disorder and severe Learning and Communication Disorders on the other, remain assessment and conceptual challenges (Harris et al., 1996; Semrud-Klikeman & Hynd, 1990). Volkmar, Klin, Marans, and McDougle (1996) suggest that the concept of Asperger's Disorder may have been broadened by its recent popularity, with a resulting overlap with PDD NOS. They suggest that a relatively stringent application of the DSM-IV (or ICD-10) criteria will help clarify the boundaries of these categories. Szatmari (1996) echoes this call for a conservative approach to diagnosis of the PDD categories, in order to achieve differentiation between the diagnoses.

Again, with the availability of Asperger's Disorder as a diagnosis, there will no doubt be more research on the boundaries of PDD that will help inform future evaluation efforts. This is an area where all professionals will need to follow the emerging literature closely. The long-term outcome of children with a diagnosis of Asperger's Disorder remains unclear.

Pervasive Developmental Disorder Not Otherwise Specified (Including Atypical Autism)

The residual category of PDD NOS remains highly heterogeneous, but with the availability of the three new specific PDD categories, the number of PDD NOS diagnoses made can be expected to be reduced from those made with the DSM-III-R criteria. Of note is that with the return of an age-of-onset criterion for Autistic Disorder, PDD NOS will be the appropriate classification of those infrequent cases that appear to meet full criteria for Autistic Disorder, but in which onset occurs after 3 years of apparently unremarkable development. With the possibility that the symptomatic presentation of Autistic Disorder may reflect a final common behavioral manifestation for several different etiologies it is likely that this will continue to be an area of active investigation. Once more, it will be important for the school psychologist to stay familiar with the emerging literature, for this is an area where remarkable advances may take place in the near future.

As noted above, distinguishing Autistic Disorder, Asperger's Disorder, and PDD NOS will represent a diagnostic challenge for the examiner, especially if there is associated lower intellectual functioning (Borderline Intellectual Functioning or very low average IQ). Collection of a careful developmental history, where possible, will settle some diagnostic questions (Volkmar, 1996). Some questionable cases will be settled with confidence only on the basis of longitudinal course, especially if a child is initially evaluated at a young age. Some cases will, in my experience, remain diagnostically unsettled; however, the number of these should be reduced by the greater differentiation of PDDs in DSM-IV.

PSYCHOSES

A second group of diagnoses that an examiner should consider when confronted with severely disturbed and disorganized maladjustment in a child or adolescent are those that have traditionally been subsumed under the heading of "psychoses." The introduction to the "Schizophrenia and Other Psychotic Disorders" chapter of DSM-IV gives a brief and clear discussion of some of the meanings that have been attached to the term "psychosis," as well as the general referents for the term in the several DSM-IV Psychotic Disorder diagnoses (p. 273): Schizophrenia, Schizophreniform Disorder, Schizoaffective Disorder, Delusional Disorder, Brief Psychotic Disorder, Shared Psychotic Disorder, Psychotic Disorder Due to a General Medical Condition, Substance-Induced Psychotic Disorder, and Psychotic Disorder NOS. (The reader interested in alternative conceptualizations may find a 1996 article by Carson stimulating as a challenge to the DSM-IV formulation of psychosis.) I discuss Psychotic Disorders below, along with a few other disorders in which psychotic symptoms may appear. The next IDEA Note sets forth how the Psychotic Disorders relate to eligibility for services under IDEA.

IDEA NOTE   Psychotic Disorders

Schizophrenia and other Psychotic Disorders in DSM-IV definitely qualify for inclusion under IDEA through the "seriously emotionally disturbed" category. A Psychotic Disorder exemplifies the basic meaning of a serious emotional disturbance, both for the general public and for members of professional disciplines involved with mental health. The disruptive symptoms and devastating life consequences of Schizophrenia and the other Psychotic Disorders easily fulfill the requirements for a handicapping condition in the IDEA legislation.

Schizophrenia and Other Psychotic Disorders

Schizophrenia

The core syndrome definition in this chapter of DSM-IV is that of Schizophrenia. Schizophrenia has been the paradigm psychotic disorder since Kraepelin's original discussion of "dementia praecox" and Bleuler's elaboration of the primary and secondary symptoms of "the schizophrenias." Schizophrenia is defined by a group of characteristic symptoms that have persisted over at least 1 month, with some continuous signs of disturbance for at least 6 months. The DSM-IV Criterion A symptom set contains both positive and negative symptoms. The DSM-IV positive symptoms (four of the five symptoms) are delusions, hallucinations, disorganized speech, and extremely disorganized or catatonic behavior. The set of negative symptoms—that is, flattening of mood, impoverished thinking, and problems with goal-directed activities—makes up the fifth criterion symptom. Anhedonia (absence of pleasure or joy) is sometimes discussed as a negative symptom, but in DSM-IV it is included only as an associated symptom. A fuller discussion of negative symptoms would have been helpful; Carpenter, Heinrichs, and Wagman (1988) provide an informative discussion of these symptoms. Additional requirements for the diagnosis of Schizophrenia include a decline in level of general adjustment (or failure to make expected developmental advances, in children and adolescents); an exclusion of Schizoaffective Disorder and of a Mood Disorder, Severe With Psychotic Features, as explanations for the problematic behaviors; and an exclusion of general medical conditions or substance use effects as the cause of the disorder. Four subtypes of Schizophrenia (Paranoid, Disorganized, Catatonic and Undifferentiated Types) are proposed. A Residual Type is also provided to cover cases of partial remission after a full-criterion episode.

There is no unique set of symptoms for childhood- or adolescent-onset Schizophrenia; the same criteria set is used for all ages. Schizophrenia usually shows an initial episode in late adolescence or early adulthood, but childhood-onset cases and early-adolescent-onset cases have been documented and can be diagnosed with the Schizophrenia criteria set (Asarnow, 1994). Werry (1996) has suggested the terms "early-onset" for Schizophrenia that develops in childhood or adolescence, and "very-early-onset" for Schizophrenia that develops before age 13; it is useful to be aware of these ideas, but DSM-IV makes no such distinctions. There are developmental features evident in childhood-onset Schizophrenia: An insidious onset is typical; there is usually a history of poor adjustment; and positive symptoms only begin to manifest themselves after the child reaches 6–9 years of age (Asarnow, 1994). About two-thirds of children who are diagnosed with Schizophrenia will also meet criteria for other mental disorders (Russell, Bott, & Sammons, 1989). The most common comorbid diagnoses are Disruptive Behavior Disorders (Conduct Disorder and Oppositional Defiant Disorder) and Depressive Disorders (Dysthymic Disorder and Depressive Disorder NOS). A careful review and consideration of possible alternative explanations should precede any application of this most serious diagnosis to a young person, but there are absolutely cases where it is indicated.

A major differential diagnosis challenge for early-onset Schizophrenia is Bipolar I Disorder. Werry (1996) suggests that Bipolar I Disorder was probably underdiagnosed in adolescents in the past and may be overdiagnosed currently in youth who show clear evidence of psychotic symptom. Based on his long-term follow-up studies of both disorders in children and adolescents, Werry (1996, p. 33) suggests the following indications favoring Schizophrenia as the more likely diagnosis: (1) long-standing premorbid abnormality, (2) psychosis lasting more than three months, (3) a deteriorating course, and (4) a family history of Schizophrenia. Werry cautions, however, that long-term follow-up is the only basis upon which to reach a firm conclusion, and advises examiners to be willing to reconsider their initial formulations in the light of additional evidence. This is sage advice with respect to all diagnostic activity with youth.

Schizophrenia can be diagnosed concurrently with Autistic Disorder or in an individual with a history of a PDD. The explicit requirement in these cases is that the symptom picture must include prominent delusions or hallucinations. It appears that the co-occurrence of Schizophrenia in children with a history of a PPD is no greater than would be expected by chance (Asarnow, 1994). The boundaries and relationships between Schizophrenia, Mood Disorders, PDDs, and other mental disorders remain an area of active investigation.

Differentiating psychotic hallucinations from other phenomena in children can be clinically challenging. Pilowsky (1986) has offered some guidelines for evaluating apparent hallucinatory behavior in children. He suggests several aspects of a case that may increase the evaluator's confidence that the child is actually experiencing perceptual distortions: (1) a spontaneous report of hallucinations (vs. material elicited by questioning); (2) vivid hallucinations (vs. reports of vague or indistinct experiences); (3) the child's belief in the reality of the hallucination (vs. reservation and doubt about the nature of the experience); (4) the child's experience that the perceptions are coming from outside the child (vs. the belief that the experiences arise from within the child him self or herself); and (5) the apparent absence of volitional control over the perceptions (vs. the ability to dismiss the voices at will). The empirical literature on hallucinations in children is limited. My own experience is that Pilowsky's characteristics may have more positive predictive power than negative predictive power. That is, the presence of the variables he believes to be associated with true hallucinations seems much more informative than their absence does. Hallucinations in children need to be distinguished from a number of normal phenomena (Pilowsky, 1986): eidetic imagery (total visual recall is much more frequent in children than in adolescents or adults), imaginary companions, and hypnogogic and hypnopompic hallucinations (vivid but normal hallucinations that occur when a child is falling asleep or just waking up).

The evaluation of both hallucinations and delusions in children depends, in part, on the children's ability to distinguish reality from imagination, fantasy, and dream. This becomes increasingly suspect if a child's mental age is less than about 6 years, and diagnostic caution is very appropriate. I would reiterate Pilowsky's caution regarding spontaneous versus elicited reports of hallucinations in children. Most children are highly suggestible to communications from most adults under many conditions; this is an empirical finding that has been robustly supported. It has been my experience with over two decades of graduate students that most examiners are relatively unaware of how leading their questions may be. In short, evaluators should regard elicited reports of hallucinations in young children with a healthy suspiciousness, in the absence of supporting evidence.

Schizophreniform Disorder

Schizophreniform Disorder is identical to Schizophrenia except for the duration of symptoms. It is, by definition, a disorder of more than 1 month but less than 6 months that meets the criterion set for Schizophrenia. The next Coding Note discusses the duration requirement for Schizophreniform Disorder in more detail.

Brief Psychotic Disorder

Brief Psychotic Disorder is defined as a brief and limited period (1 day to 1 month) of at least one positive symptom of psychosis (delusions, hallucinations, disorganized speech, or extremely disorganized or catatonic behavior). The specifier With Marked Stressor(s) is available, but a major stressor is not required for the diagnosis. With Post-

CODING NOTE   Schizophreniform Disorder in Children
and Adolescents

> If a young person who shows symptoms meeting the criterion set for
> Schizophrenia (except for duration of symptoms) recovers in less than
> 6 months, then the correct diagnosis is Schizophreniform Disorder. If
> the young person does not recover, but 6 months have not yet passed,
> then the correct diagnosis is Schizophreniform Disorder (Provisional).
> If the disorder persists longer than 6 months the diagnosis should be
> changed to Schizophrenia. The course and duration of the disturbance
> are critical diagnostic elements in assigning the correct DSM-IV diag-
> nosis for a Psychotic Disorder.

partum Onset is also available as a specifier, the diagnosis of Brief
Psychotic Disorder is not made if the symptoms are better accounted
for by a Mood Disorder. Careful evaluation is necessary to exclude
psychotic symptoms resulting from general medical conditions or use
of a substance (medication, toxin, or drug of abuse).

The major difference among Brief Psychotic Disorder, Schizophreniform Disorder, and Schizophrenia involves duration of disturbance: 1 day to 1 month, 1 month to 6 months, and more than 6
months, respectively.

Schizoaffective Disorder

Schizoaffective Disorder reflects a disturbance that concurrently meets
the criteria both for Schizophrenia and for a Major Depressive, Manic,
or Mixed Episode of mood symptoms. This can be a confusing diagnostic category, both conceptually and in actual practice. Mood symptoms, especially depression and anhedonia, are common associated
symptoms in individuals with Schizophrenia or another Psychotic
Disorder. Furthermore, pure Mood Disorders (both Major Depressive Disorder and Bipolar I and II Disorders) can exacerbate to the
point of psychosis (see "Additional Diagnostic Categories Involving
Psychosis," below. The diagnosis of Schizoaffective Disorder, however,
is not made in cases involving isolated symptoms, but in cases meeting full criteria for both a Mood Episode (Major Depressive, Manic,
or Mixed) and the core symptoms of Schizophrenia simultaneously.

Very careful documentation of history is required to establish
this diagnosis with any confidence, and this necessity is complicated

by the clinical state of an affected individual (young people with Psychotic Disorders are not usually reliable historians). After the psychotic symptoms have begun to clear or respond to treatment, the client may be more responsive to interviewing, but may not remember the information of interest because of the cognitive disruption produced by the psychotic episode. My experience has been that only the use of multiple informants who have had regular contact with the individual over the course of his or her problems yields diagnostic confidence with respect to this diagnosis. The next Coding Note presents further reflections on Schizoaffective Disorder.

Delusional Disorder

Delusional Disorder (Paranoia in DSM-III, Delusional [Paranoid] Disorder in DSM-III-R) is a Psychotic Disorder involving prominent delusions without other prominent symptoms of psychosis. The delusions must be nonbizarre. The individual can have no history of Schizophrenia. This disorder is not usually seen in adolescents or children.

Shared Psychotic Disorder (Folie à Deux)

Shared Psychotic Disorder reflects a delusion that is acquired through a long-standing, intimate relationship with an individual who has a primary Psychotic Disorder with prominent delusions. The special circumstances necessary here obviously limit the prevalence of this possibility, but cases involving children do occur. Children may come

---

CODING NOTE   Schizoaffective Disorder in Children and Adolescents

If a child or adolescent concurrently shows full symptoms for both Schizophrenia and a Mood Episode (Major Depressive, Manic, or Mixed), then the correct DSM-IV diagnosis is Schizoaffective Disorder. The boundaries and relationships between affective disorders and thought disorders continue to be actively debated and investigated. In my experience, the clinical population identified with a classification of Schizoaffective Disorder remains highly heterogeneous, with some clients presenting with more Mood Disorder qualities and others with more features of Schizophrenia or other Psychotic Disorders. Further work may result in significant revision of the category.

---

to believe and be willing to discuss freely the delusional thoughts of a psychotic parent. The initial contact with such a family may be occasioned by clinical interest in a child or adolescent who has voiced ideas at school that have aroused concern. Only in following up with the family may it become apparent that the young person is merely echoing the beliefs of a parent with a Psychotic Disorder.

This unusual category can raise difficult questions of therapeutic management. In a case I saw early in my training, a single mother brought her three daughters into a public clinic for vaccinations. The attending resident became concerned over the "crazy ideas" voiced by the two younger girls. When I sat down with their mother to share our concerns about her daughters, it became apparent that she fully shared (and was probably the origin of) their delusions. An interview with the third and oldest daughter revealed that she too acknowledged the family's unique thoughts, but was very reticent about sharing these with the examiner; her public behavior appeared to have come under contingency control by the broader community she interacted with. The case caused some debate among the professionals involved. The young mother appeared to be clearly delusional and to have taught her children to be delusional; at the same time this case had only come to our attention because this mother was very responsible with respect to the medical needs of her children (in the city we served, a disturbing percentage of residents had not obtained the recommended health checks and vaccinations for their children). Furthermore, there was no evidence that the children were neglected or abused. Their medical health was unremarkable. They appeared well fed and clothed, happy and unafraid, positively attached to their caretaker—and delusional. The oldest child showed evidence of having learned to be circumspect about sharing family ideas with outsiders. With the young mother's consent, we communicated with her parents; the parents, we learned, were aware of their daughter's mental health history and communicated regularly with her psychiatrist.

Other Psychotic Disorders

Psychotic Disorder Due to a General Medical Condition and Substance-Induced Psychotic Disorder reflect psychotic symptoms (delusions and/or hallucinations without insight) associated with specific, established etiologies. Both should be actively evaluated as possibilities in the assessment of acute psychotic symptoms in a young person, especially in the absence of a family history of severe mental health problems. Even in an adolescent with a history of a primary Psychotic Disorder, the possibility of a Substance-Induced Psychotic Disorder should be aggressively considered if there is anything about the circumstances that does not seem consistent with the youth's history. Adolescents, including young people with atypical perceptual processing, are at some risk for substance experimentation. Individuals at risk for Schizophrenia may be especially vulnerable to intense, unpleasant, and/or idiosyncratic reactions to drugs of abuse. Comorbid presentations of Substance Use Disorders and Psychotic Disorders are unfortunately familiar to most mental health workers dealing with adolescents and young adults.

Psychotic Disorder NOS covers a variety of residual cases where there is evidence of psychotic symptomatology but the data necessary to make a more specific diagnosis are lacking or conflicted. Various descriptive labels have appeared in the clinical literature to identify individuals who show mixed symptom presentations of thought disorders, affective disorders, language disorders, and hyperactivity. Barkley (1990) has discussed children with problems he calls "multiplex developmental disorders"; Rapoport (1997) has discussed a group of children she refers to as "multidimensionally impaired." In some cases, Psychotic Disorder NOS will be resolved into a more specific diagnosis as further information is collected and/or the course of the disorder unfolds. The next Coding Note presents guidelines for distinguishing between Psychotic Disorder NOS and Brief Psychotic Disorder.

Comorbid and Premorbid Disorders

Epidemiological data suggest that poor childhood adjustment may be a premorbid risk factor for some of the Psychotic Disorders. Along with the many other negative prognostic associations for Conduct

---

CODING NOTE   Psychotic Disorder NOS
   and Brief Psychotic Disorder

Psychotic Disorder NOS is the appropriate classification when a case may turn out to meet the criteria for a diagnosis of Brief Psychotic Disorder, but the symptoms have not yet remitted (psychotic symptoms have lasted for more than 1 day and less than 1 month, but are still present). If the psychotic symptoms do eventually remit in less than 1 month, the diagnosis should be changed from Psychotic Disorder NOS to Brief Psychotic Disorder. (See also the Coding Note on p. 159.)

Disorder is an overrepresentation among adult populations with psychotic diagnoses. Substance Abuse and (less frequently) Substance Dependence are other comorbid problems for individuals with Schizophrenia.

The three Cluster A Personality Disorders (Schizotypal, Schizoid, Paranoid) have been hypothesized to be associated premorbidly with one or more of the Psychotic Disorders. This remains an issue of contention and ongoing interest, but it is certainly of value to attempt to elicit any reliable information possible on premorbid adjustment and personality traits in youth diagnosed with a Psychotic Disorder. The three Cluster A Personality Disorders are only made as comorbid diagnoses of Schizophrenia and other Psychotic Disorders if there is clear evidence that the personality pattern occurs at times other than acute psychotic episodes.

Additional Diagnostic Categories Involving Psychosis

Several Mood Disorders can reach such severity that psychotic symptoms appear. The specifier Severe With Psychotic Features can be used for Major Depressive Episodes that occur in the course of Major Depressive, Bipolar I, and Bipolar II Disorders, as well as for Manic and Mixed Episodes that occur in the course of Bipolar I Disorder. A table on page 376 of DSM-IV gives a summary of this and other episode specifiers applying to different Mood Disorders.

Brief and transient psychotic symptoms (hallucinations, delusions, ideas of reference, severely regressed or catatonic behavior) are often mentioned in the context of Borderline Personality Disorder in the general psychological literature. These florid manifestations are typically a reaction to extreme environmental stress (e.g., loss of an important relationship, feedback devaluating the client, rejection). DSM-III-R included transient psychotic symptoms as possible associated symptoms of this Personality Disorder. DSM-IV describes these more conservatively as "psychotic-like symptoms" (p. 652). In any event, the possible "psychotic symptoms" of Borderline Personality Disorder are relatively easily distinguished from those of the Psychotic Disorders proper by their brevity and predictable relationship to situational events.

◆

See DSM-IV-TR Coding Note: Pervasive Developmental Disorder NOS in DSM-IV-TR, in 2002 Updates, page 237.

CHAPTER 10

Personality Disorders

♦

DIAGNOSING PERSONALITY DISORDERS IN YOUTH: CONTROVERSY AND CAUTIONS

The question of whether Personality Disorders actually occur in children and adolescents is a relatively new one and has generated a certain amount of controversy. The basic idea of a "personality disorder" is of a sustained pattern of rigid and excessive traits that compromises an individual's adjustment or functioning. The construct of "personality" is, of course, a very old one in psychology, and its study has reflected the various concerns of groups within the social sciences. The idea that there are reliable, cross-situational consistencies in actions was challenged by some social learning theorists during the 1970s (Mischel, 1968), but in more recent formulations may behavioral theorists seem to accept some degree of consistency in human behavior, paralleling conventional ideas of personality. Cognitive-behavioral treatment approaches for Personality Disorders have further established this renewed acceptance of the concept of personality (Beck, Freeman, & Associates, 1990; Linehan, 1993; Turkat, 1990; Young, 1990), although a few behavioral theorists still do not accept the concept's usefulness (see, e.g., Koerner, Kohlenberg, & Parker, 1996).

DSM-IV defines "personality traits" as "enduring patterns of perceiving, relating to, and thinking about the environment and oneself that are exhibited in a wide range of social and personal contexts" (p. 630). A Personality Disorder is characterized by traits that are inflexible, are maladaptive, and cause either significant personality distress or functional impairment (the fundamental criterion for a mental disorders). The dysfunctional pattern of a Personality Disorder must be evident across a range of environmental settings, consistent and enduring over time, and evident by adolescence or early adulthood. From this basic view of personality problems emerges the confict inherent in using the Personality Disorder categories with children and adolescents. Explicit in the very definition of a Personality Disorder is the belief that these excessively rigid traits should be manifested from relatively early in life (and should therefore be available for clinical diagnosis). Yet, from a different perspective, it can be questioned how much confidence we can ever have in a Personality Disorder diagnosis in childhood or adolescence. To what extent has there been any opportunity to evaluate how stable this behavior pattern will be across settings when a young person has usually experienced relatively few environments? And how can we speak of stability over time when the young person has lived but a small fraction of his or her potential life-span? A few empirical data on use of the DSM-III-R Personality Disorder diagnoses with youth have become available (see Bernstein et al., 1993), but a great deal of additional work will be necessary before the clinical and empirical acceptability of these diagnoses with youth is established. Probably the best empirical case for the stability and validity of a Personality Disorder category applied to children and youth could be made for Antisocial Personality Disorder—which, as it happens, is the *only* Personality Disorder diagnosis explicitly precluded from use when the client is less than 18 years of age.

With the exception of Antisocial Personality Disorder, the Personality Disorder diagnoses (which, of course, are coded on Axis II; see the following Coding Note) are available for use with older children and adolescents. DSM-IV requires only that the diagnostic features must have been evident for at least 1 year in clients under 18 years of age (p. 631). My own recommendation, however, is for caution in using Personality Disorder diagnoses in youth (see also Lewis, 1996). Although indicating dysfunctional personality traits may be very useful in understanding the problems of a young person, and

---

CODING NOTE   Personality Disorders and Axis II

In DSM-IV the Personality Disorders remain on Axis II, where they were in DSM-III and DSM-III-R. As noted elsewhere in this book, only the Personality Disorders have consistently been placed on Axis II across the three presentations of DSM as a multiaxial diagnostic system.

---

may set very valuable targets for therapeutic change, the decision to conceptualize the problems of a very young person as a Personality Disorder implies a stability that I believe is often lacking in the reactions of individuals during their first quarter-century of life. I would advise that as part of making a decision about use of a Personality Disorder diagnosis, examiners should consider not only the specific categorical criteria, but also the general diagnostic criteria for a Personality Disorder (p. 635). I believe that a useful heuristic is frequently patience: If a young person actually has a Personality Disorder, then the problems will continue, and even more evidence of the disorder's existence will accumulate. This does not mean that therapeutic efforts to enhance the young person's adjustment need be postponed. The evaluator can identify problematic behavior patterns and make these the focus of change efforts. If the behavior problems are resistant to these efforts, the case for a Personality Disorder is strengthened; if moderation is achieved and a better level of adjustment and functioning results, then the question is moot.

OTHER CAUTIONS ABOUT DIAGNOSING PERSONALITY DISORDERS

DSM-IV recommends caution in diagnosing Personality Disorders during active episodes of Mood or Anxiety Disorders, because the symptoms of these disorders may "mimic" personality traits and may complicate the retrospective evaluation of a client's long-standing temperament. This caution seems well advised. The cognitive features associated with mood and anxiety problems may distort retrospective reports, and it is possible that the experience of interacting with a depressed adolescent or child may influence the retrospective impression of a caretaker who is being interviewed about "premorbid personality features." Although the possibility of personality traits and potentially dysfunctional personality traits can always be noted on Axis II, I would recommend that Personality Disorders not be based exclusively on data gathered during acute episodes of Mood, Anxiety, Somatoform, or Dissociative Disorders.

Another consideration that must be given especial attention in the potential diagnosis of a Personality Disorder is any potential involvement in substance misuse. The literature on the reliability of Personality Disorder diagnoses in adults strongly suggests the hazard of making such diagnoses during periods of active Substance Abuse or Dependence, or during detoxification from Substance Dependence. In the absence of clear evidence of years of premorbid occurrence of rigid and dysfunctional personality traits prior to any active substance use by a child or adolescent, I would recommend deferring any diagnosis of a Personality Disorder until after establishment of a stable period of substance free living. Nevertheless, significant associations have been reported between Substance Use Disorders and Borderline Personality Disorder (BPD) in adolescents, and especially among Substance Use Disorders, Major Depressive Disorders, and BPD (Grilo, Walker, Becker, Edell, & McGlashan, 1997).

Personality Disorder diagnoses on Axis II are frequently, and possibly usually, associated with comorbid Axis I diagnoses (Lewinsohn, Rohde, Seeley, & Klein, 1997). Personality Disorder diagnoses are associated with greater distress and functional impairment in troubled adolescents (Bernstein et al., 1993). Finally, although some adolescent diagnoses of Personality Disorder are stable over time, many were not found to be evident at the end of a 2-year follow-up study (Bernstein et al., 1993). Considering the multiple indications that personality phenomena may be better conceptualized as traits than as types, there may be inherent limitations in a categorical model of personality pattern difficulty.

Given these preliminary considerations, let us now consider the three broad groupings of Personality Disorders within DSM-IV: Cluster A (odd–eccentric), Cluster B (dramatic–emotional), and Cluster C (anxious–fearful). The next IDEA Note sets forth how Personality Disorders in general and the Cluster B disorders in particular relate to eligibility for services under IDEA.

CLUSTER A (ODD–ECCENTRIC) PERSONALITY DISORDERS

With the exception of Antisocial Personality Disorder, which by definition shows a childhood or young adolescent precursor state (i.e., Conduct Disorder), possibly the best evidence for the existence of Personality Disorder phenomena in youth can be marshaled for the categories from the odd–eccentric cluster of Personality Disorders: Paranoid, Schizoid, and Schizotypal Personality Disorders. All are described as possibly being first apparent in childhood, with similar manifestations and social consequences (peer rejection, teasing). A discussion of the role of this social isolation from possibly "corrective" peer feedback in the possible exacerbation of these problems is beyond the scope of this work, but it is clearly an area for further investigation. The available literature suggests that all three patterns in their extreme (i.e., diagnosable) form may be very stable. This is

IDEA NOTE Personality Disorders and IDEA

I am unaware of any cases where eligibility for special services under IDEA has been sought on the basis of a diagnosed Personality Disorder in a child or adolescent. Given the high reported comorbidity of Axis I disorders in youth classified as manifesting Personality Disorders, it is likely that there are young people with Personality Disorders who are receiving special education or other services, but that their eligibility was demonstrated on the basis of the Axis I disorders. Nevertheless, given the very disruptive nature of the Cluster B (dramatic–emotional) Personality Disorders it is quite possible that one may eventually be identified as the primary or sole reason for a young person's need of services under IDEA. The very nature of Personality Disorders—enduring, resistant to change, rigid, and nonadaptive—should address most of the basic requirements of the "seriously emotionally disturbed" category of eligibility.

The essential task of the school psychologist advancing such a case will be to demonstrate the functional limitations manifested in the child's or adolescent's school performance because of these characteristics. This may or may not pose a challenge. For some young people with personality trait disturbances, the interference with their school achievement is evident to all observers. Yet it has been my experience that some adolescents showing borderline traits may actually do their best in academic activities. The structure and attention available in schoolwork may help them constrain their rigid and extreme temperament and achieve a degree of confidence and success not seen in other areas of their lives. The ongoing discussion of including social maladjustment problems in IDEA should bring even more attention to this question of how Personality Disorders should be treated under IDEA.

---

an especially interesting conclusion regarding Schizotypal Personality Disorder, which was originally conceptualized as a possible precursor to Schizophrenia. DSM-IV points out the potential difficulty in distinguishing Schizoid Personality Disorder from Asperger's Disorder and from milder manifestations of Autistic Disorder. The differentiation is based on severity of social impairments and restricted repertoire. Although the general cautions about using Personality Disorder diagnoses with children and adolescents (discussed above) also apply to the Cluster A categories, these would seem to constitute an area of both valid clinical use and continued empirical investigation.

CLUSTER B (DRAMATIC–EMOTIONAL) PERSONALITY DISORDERS

Antisocial Personality Disorder

As noted above, Antisocial Personality Disorder cannot be diagnosed prior to age 18; by definition, however, there is preexisting Conduct Disorder before the age of 15. I have found it valuable to note in adolescent classifications those cases where continuation of the observed pattern of antisocial behavior will justify a clinical diagnosis of Antisocial Personality Disorder when the individuals reach the age of 18.

Borderline Personality Disorder

The usefulness of conceptualizing difficult-to-deal-with youth as manifesting BPD will undoubtedly continue to be actively debated (Bleiberg, 1994; Lewis, 1996), especially as validated treatments for BPD become available (Linehan, 1993). In my experience, this is the Personality Disorder category most commonly evoked in classifying adolescents—especially those with chronic problems, poor response to treatments, and demanding personality features. Yet, despite concern over heterogeneity of populations, the possibility that "borderline" characteristics or even diagnoses of BPD in children are not good predictors of BPD in adults (Lewis, 1996), and worry that we may be doing little more than applying a prejudicial label to particularly troublesome clients, there is some evidence that BPD may be a viable diagnostic category for adolescents (Ludolph et al., 1990; Westen, Ludolph, Lerner, Ruffins, & Wiss, 1990). A study by Guzder, Paris, Zelkowitz, and Marchessault (1996) on risk factors for borderline pathology in children is worth considering; this group found that sexual abuse, physical abuse, severe neglect, and parental Substance Abuse or criminal behavior differentiated between their groups of children with and without a diagnosis of BPD (made with the Child Diagnostic Interview for Borderlines). The Grilo et al. (1997) study cited above reported higher rates of BPD in hospitalized adolescents with diagnoses of Major Depressive Disorder, with diagnoses of a Substance Use Disorder, and especially with a combination of Major Depressive Disorder and a Substance Use Disorder.

I have sometimes found it useful to identify borderline traits being displayed by an adolescent. These can be identified, listed, or discussed (but not coded) on Axis II. I have had very few occasions to feel confident about applying a DSM-IV diagnosis of BPD to an adolescent, however. Goldman, D'Angelo, Demaso, and Mezzacappa (1992) suggested modifications of the DSM-III-R criterion set for BPD to make it more applicable to adolescents. I believe the best course if a teenager is identified by such a modified criterion set, but does not meet the DSM-IV criteria, is to make a diagnosis of Personality Disorder NOS and explain that the young person does meet an experimental set of diagnostic criteria. I would still advise great caution regarding the utility of a conceptualization of BPD in adolescents, because this diagnosis in youth seems to be more strongly associated with Axis I diagnoses than with an Axis II diagnosis follow-up (Lewis, 1996).

Another diagnostic concern is that multiple Axis I mental disorders may occur in association with BPD. Concurrent Mood Disorders, Anxiety Disorders, Substance Use Disorders, Attention-Deficit/Hyperactivity Disorder, Conduct Disorder, and (in a few cases) Dissociative Disorders may occur. The combination of BPD with Depressive Disorders may be especially dangerous with respect to suicide risk (Pfeffer, 1992). Repeated instances of nonlethal, self-injurious behaviors are almost pathognomonic for BPD (Linehan, 1993), but some care must be exercised to differentiate between these and various subculturally supported "deviant behaviors of youth"—nonprofessional tattooing, body piercing, decorative scarring, and the like, which can also be seen both in youth with Conduct Disorders and in extremely rebellious or idiosyncratic (but not mentally ill) youth.

Histrionic Personality Disorder

DSM-IV offers no specific information on the use of the Histrionic Personality Disorder category in youth. The manual's general caution, however, is well considered: "Many individuals may display histrionic personality traits. Only when these traits are inflexible, maladaptive, and persisting and cause significant functional impairment or subjective distress do they constitute Histrionic Personality Disorder" (p. 657).

Narcissistic Personality Disorder

DSM-IV notes only that narcissistic traits are common during adolescence and do not predict the development of Narcissistic Personality Disorder. Although pathological narcissistic traits probably develop in childhood and adolescence, I have not found this to be a useful Personality Disorder diagnosis in youth. Noting apparently extreme narcissistic traits on Axis II can be helpful in case conceptualization and management.

CLUSTER C (ANXIOUS–FEARFUL)
PERSONALITY DISORDERS

Avoidant Personality Disorder

DSM-IV recommends caution in using the Avoidant Personality Disorder diagnosis with children and adolescents, because shy and avoidant behavior may be both typical and developmentally appropriate. The available literature on avoidant personality problems suggest that these usually do begin in childhood, when stranger shyness is common; however, in the typical developmental course these excessive fear reactions decrease with social experience, whereas the problems increase with age and experience for the individual who will eventually be labeled as having Avoidant Personality Disorder. Sensitivity to this potential problem of youth is well advised.

DSM-IV points out in its discussion of differential diagnosis that Social Phobia, Generalized Type overlaps in symptomatic presentation with Avoidant Personality Disorder to a great extent; indeed, these two categories may be two different conceptualizations of the same difficulty. Social Phobia will often serve as an accurate diagnosis of a child who shows severe avoidant traits, and such a diagnosis will avoid the difficulties inherent in using Personality Disorder diagnoses with children.

Dependent Personality Disorder

DSM-IV also recommends great caution in the use of the Dependent Personality Disorder category with children and adolescents, because a dependent pattern is developmentally normal and appropriate. If the presenting problems involve functioning apart from the caretaker, the Axis I category of Separation Anxiety Disorder should be considered. I have noted dependent traits in children and adolescents, but have never used this Personality Disorder diagnosis with youth.

Obsessive–Compulsive Personality Disorder

DSM-IV offers no information regarding the use of the Obsessive–Compulsive Personality Disorder category with children and adolescents. I have encountered no clinical cases of its use in my professional practice. A common mistake is the confusion of Obsessive–Compulsive Personality Disorder with Obsessive–Compulsive Disorder. The Axis I category involves specific symptoms (obsessions or compulsions), whereas the Personality Disorder pattern "is a preoccupation with orderliness, perfectionism, and mental and interpersonal control, at the expense of flexibility, openness, and efficiency" (p. 669). Despite the common elements in their labels (reflecting a previous belief in common psychodynamic features), the available evidence does not suggest an empirical linkage of these two problems. Adults with Obsessive–Compulsive Personality Disorder do not seem especially prone to manifest Obsessive Compulsive Disorders as well; nor is Obsessive–Compulsive Personality Disorder commonly reported in individuals who present with Obsessive–Compulsive Disorder.

RESIDUAL CASES

The Personality Disorder Not Otherwise Specified category is provided for cases that do meet the general criteria for a Personality Disorder (p. 633), but do not meet the criteria for one of the delineated DSM-IV categories. The two general examples discussed briefly are (1) a "mixed personality," which shows features of more than one specific Personality Disorder pattern, but does not meet full criteria for any one; and (2) the perception of a specific pattern of trait dysfunction not formally recognized by DSM-IV. Included in Appendix B, "Criteria Sets and Axes Provided for Further Study," are proposed criterion sets for two categories: dependent personality disorder and passive–aggressive personality disorder. Depressive personality disorder is a new proposed category (but certainly not a new concept), and distinguishing it from Dysthymic Disorder would seem problematic. For children and adolescents, I would strongly suggest consideration of Dysthymic Disorder as an appropriate diagnosis in most cases where depressive personality disorder is being considered. Passive–aggressive personality disorder (negativistic personality disorder) was included in the main text of DSM-III and DSM-III-R, but has been dropped from the DSM-IV classification because the empirical literature has not supported its usefulness. The champions of this historical conceptualization have managed to have it included in Appendix B. The discussion notes its similarity to Oppositional Defiant Disorder, but states that the proposed category "should only be considered in adults" (p. 734). This is excellent advice; I would not recommend the use of this diagnosis for children or adolescents. The ICD-9-CM coding for any of these residual cases—mixed, proposed, or unique cases—is the same: 301.9.

CHAPTER 11

♦♦♦

Additional Codes and Categories

♦

BROADER-BAND RESIDUAL CATEGORIES

One of the strengths of the DSM-IV classification system has been the creation of a more comprehensive set of categories with the flexibility to cover meaningfully most of the situations that confront professional psychologists and other mental health practitioners. One aspect of this, already discussed several times, has been the expansion of the Not Otherwise Specified (NOS) residual categories to include most of the thematic groups of diagnoses in DSM-IV. In addition to these focused NOS categories, there are two even broader-band diagnoses: Disorder of Infancy, Childhood, or Adolescence NOS, and Unspecified Mental Disorder (nonpsychotic). Both diagnoses are Mental Disorders; that is, the examiner's conclusion in using either one is that a case meets the basic definition of a Mental Disorder within DSM-IV. However, the examiner's conclusion is also either that the case does not meet the criteria for a diagnosis in any of the more focused areas of problem behavior, or that inadequate information is available to indicate whether the case does meet criteria for a more specific category.

Disorder of Infancy, Childhood, or Adolescence Not Otherwise Specified

Disorder of Infancy, Childhood, or Adolescence NOS is found at the end of the first content chapter of DSM-IV, "Disorders Usually First Diagnosed in Infancy, Childhood, or Adolescence." It is a residual diagnosis for disorders with a developmental onset that do not meet the criteria for any specific disorder in DSM-IV. I have neither used this category nor seen it used; however, there could be circumstances, (especially very early in an evaluation) in which it could be an appropriate working diagnosis. Use of this category indicates that the examiner has enough data to conclude the following: (1) A mental disorder is present, and (2) the mental disorder began during the first two decades of life, but (3) the available information does not allow specification within any of the content areas of DSM-IV (e.g., Disruptive Behavior Disorder NOS or Mood Disorder NOS). Presumably, further assessment will lead to a more specific diagnosis unless a truly novel pattern of maladjustment has been found.

Unspecified Mental Disorder (Nonpsychotic)

Unspecified Mental Disorder (nonpsychotic) is found on page 687 of DSM-IV, in a brief chapter titled "Additional Codes." It covers cases where the examiner can decide the following: (1) A mental disorder is present; (2) there are no signs or symptoms of psychosis; (3) either a specific behavioral pattern is identified that is not covered by DSM-IV, or insufficient data are available to make a decision about the specific pattern of problems; and (4) none of the available NOS categories are applicable. If, for instance, the client is a child or adolescent, then the diagnosis of Disorder of Infancy, Childhood, or Adolescence NOS will take precedence over Unspecified Mental Disorder (nonpsychotic) because it carries at least a little additional information.

NO DIAGNOSIS/DIAGNOSIS DEFERRED CATEGORIES

Also found in the "Additional Codes" chapter of DSM-IV are four other valuable categories: No Diagnosis on Axis I, Diagnosis Deferred on Axis I, No Diagnosis on Axis II, and Diagnosis Deferred on Axis II. The next Coding Note describes the ICD-9-CM coding for these categories.

No Diagnosis or Condition on Axis I/No Diagnosis on Axis II

The two No Diagnosis categories are positive, affirmative statements. That is, the school psychologist has evaluated a young person and his or her situation, and has concluded that a mental disorder is not present on Axis I or Axis II (or both). There may be problems in the

---

**CODING NOTE   Duplicate Codes on Axes I and II for the
No Diagnosis/Diagnosis Deferred Categories**

The ICD-9-CM code for Diagnosis or Condition Deferred on Axis I is
the same as that for Diagnosis Deferred on Axis II (799.9). Also, the
ICD-9-CM code for No Diagnosis or Condition on Axis I is the same as
that for No Diagnosis on Axis II (V71.09).

---

young person's life or with his or her behavior, but these problems
fall short of the definition of a mental disorder. Typically, the Global
Assessment of Functioning rating on Axis V in such a case is relatively
high (70 or above), but there are exceptions to this.

Diagnosis or Condition Deferred on Axis I/Diagnosis Deferred on Axis II

The two Diagnosis Deferred categories are statements of doubt. That
is, the examiner is unwilling to conclude whether a mental disorder
is present or not. Such a diagnosis is not an answer; it is a statement
that more time is needed to gather data so that a firmer conclusion
can be drawn.

APPENDIX B: PROPOSED CATEGORIES AND AXES

A final set of diagnostic categories the school psychologist needs to
be aware of is found in Appendix B of DSM-IV, "Criteria Sets and
Axes Provided for Further Study." These are proposed categories and
other functional assessments that appear to have sufficient merit to
justify investigation but are not included in the main text of DSM-IV.
A few of these categories have already been discussed earlier in the
present book. In almost every case where such a category is used, the
diagnosis should be formally coded as the NOS category in the appropriate DSM-IV chapter. The provision of criterion sets for these
patterns should help stimulate research and generate a data base that
will support (or reject) their inclusion in DSM-V or some future revision.

Criterion sets for 14 proposed diagnostic categories are given, as
well as an alternative set of dimensions to subclassify Schizophrenia
and an alternative set of symptoms (Criterion B) for Dysthymic Disor-

der (see the next Coding Note). Whereas most of these categories are new proposals, one, passive–aggressive personality disorder (negativistic personality disorder), was actually included as a personality disorder in DSM-III and DSM-III-R. Despite its venerable history in some theoretical and psychotherapeutic approaches, inadequate empirical research was found to support this classification. The movement of this category to Appendix B appears to represent a political compromise between its supporters and those who would have

---

CODING NOTE   Proposed Diagnostic Categories in Appendix B

Postconcussional disorder (should be coded as Cognitive Disorder NOS)

Mild neurocognitive disorder (should be coded as Cognitive Disorder NOS)

Caffeine withdrawal (should be coded as Caffeine-Related Disorder NOS)

Alternative dimensional descriptors for Schizophrenia

Postpsychotic depressive disorder of Schizophrenia (should be coded as Depressive Disorder NOS)

Simple deteriorative disorder (simple Schizophrenia) (should be coded as Unspecified Mental Disorder)

Premenstrual dysphoric disorder (should be coded as Depressive Disorder NOS)

Alternative Criterion B for Dysthymic Disorder

Minor depressive disorder (should be coded as Adjustment Disorder With Depressed Mood if in response to a psychosocial stressor, or as Depressive Disorder NOS in absence of identified stressor)

Recurrent brief depressive disorder (should be coded as Depressive Disorder NOS)

Mixed anxiety–depressive disorder (should be coded as Anxiety Disorder NOS)

Factitious disorder by proxy (should be coded as Factitious Disorder NOS)

Dissociative trance disorder (should be coded as Dissociative Disorder NOS)

Binge-eating disorder (should be coded as Eating Disorder NOS)

Depressive personality disorder (should be coded as Personality Disorder NOS on Axis II)

Passive–aggressive personality disorder (negativistic personality disorder) (should be coded as Personality Disorder NOS on Axis II)

---

dropped it entirely. Research criteria sets are also proposed for seven categories of Medication-Induced Movement Disorders. However, these categories are not mental disorders; they are already listed in the "Other Conditions That May Be a Focus of Clinical Attention" chapter.

In addition to the specific diagnostic categories that are provided for investigation, Appendix B contains three proposed new axes of information on coping and functional adjustment. One, the Defensive Functioning Scale, has had support previously but has not achieved complete acceptance within DSM-III, DSM-III-R, or DSM-IV. The other two proposed axes are a Global Assessment of Relational Functioning Scale and a Social and Occupational Functioning Assessment Scale. The future status of these proposed axes, as well as the proposed categories, will depend on research efforts over the years leading up to DSM-V.

PART III

THE APPLICATION OF DSM-IV IN SCHOOL SETTINGS: ISSUES AND TOPICS

◆

In teaching evaluation courses to graduate students, I have found that one of the most important tasks has been helping them understand the difference between psychological testing and psychological assessment. Testing is an essentially mechanical process that can be taught with relative ease and simplicity. I am convinced that even the most challenging of psychological tests—from the perspective of the tasks required of the examiner—could be taught adequately to high school graduates with average intelligence. Psychological assessment, by contrast, is a highly demanding, professional-level task requiring an understanding of human problems, awareness of issues in accurate testing; knowledge of the characteristics of available approaches to evaluation and characteristics of available instruments; and the integration of all this understanding and knowledge in the individual case to generate an evaluation approach that can answer the referral questions. It follows from this that psychiatric classification involves more than memorizing a set of diagnostic criteria. In most cases, I discourage my students from even trying to memorize DSM criterion sets. What evaluators need is an understanding of the process of human evaluation, thorough familiarity with (though not rote knowledge of) the classification system to be used, and a thoughtful selection of the most appropriate diagnostic codes. Like most other human activity, the process of psychiatric classification interacts with many other systems of behavior, codes of ethics and values, and people. In this final section, several topics related to the competent and professional use of DSM-IV in the classification of emotional and behavioral problems in children are considered.

CHAPTER 12

♦♦♦

Ethics and Professional Responsibility in Evaluation

♦

THE ROLE OF THE SCHOOL PSYCHOLOGIST IN MENTAL HEALTH ASSESSMENT

The issue of which professions should be involved in making emotional and behavioral classifications is a complicated one, probably with both rational and less than rational elements. There is a lack of consensus even over what the activity should be called: "psychiatric diagnosis," "mental health assessment," "behavioral diagnosis," or the like. Professional pride and vanity, legal definitions of medical and psychological practice, discipline/guild issues of professional autonomy and economic competition, and the social forces that have shaped and reshaped mental health practice in the 20th century have all played a role. The broad topic of psychology as an independent profession is well beyond the scope of this text, but the specific question of what role school psychologists should play in behavioral classification is important.

Psychologists have long been involved in the classification of behavioral and emotional disorders. One obvious area of this involvement has been psychological testing within mental health services. Testing was for a long period the special province of psychologists, and to the degree that testing proved valuable to the process of evaluation, psychologists were drawn into this process (despite any contrary opinions). For the intellectual, academic, and cognitive disorders, the role of formal psychometric assessment is often primary. Very few professionals of any discipline would attempt to diagnose mental retardation, learning disabilities, or dementia without formal ability testing. The contributions of behavior rating scales to the evaluation of many childhood problems, symptom report scales to the assessment of mood and anxiety problems, and global measures of temperament and social relationships to models of personality dysfunction are all well documented. One could well argue that the extensive preparation in assessment that is a part of most psychology training programs places psychologists in an optimal position for making reliable and valid assessments of patterns of maladjustment. Clinical and counseling psychologists in a wide range of professional settings are routinely called upon to make classifications of their clients within the format of DSM-IV.

School psychologists have been no less involved in the assessment and description of behavior and behavior problems than psychologists in other applied specialities have been. Their work traditions, however, have often not involved expressing these evaluations in the language of a psychiatric classification system. The highly competent assessments of school psychologists have usually been aimed at establishing young persons' eligibility for special services within the educational system, helping to plan individualized educational programs, or monitoring change and progress over the course of young people's educational career. Even the first of these functions has generally been carried out in the context of a very different and specialized classification system, developed within and largely restricted to school settings and educational purposes. The psychological assessments of most school psychologists have contained data based on behavioral observations, psychological testing, historical records, and the report of significant others in a child's or adolescent's life; but not usually any expression of how this information would be represented within the DSM-IV classification system. Until recently, this has not been viewed as part of the role of the school psychologist.

Numerous influences, however, have begun to change this state of affairs. School psychologists and the educational systems that employ them are increasingly asking whether psychiatric classification should be part of the school psychologists' role. One obviously powerful factor is economics. Mental health diagnosis makes available the possibility of accessing other potential sources of funding for psychological services within schools—the "third-party payers" of insurance companies, as well as of state and federal government agencies. With increasing legislative mandates to provide an ever-enlarging range of services, often without any corresponding additional funding, schools are being pressed to the limits of their financial resources. Some have begun exploring the possibility of accessing commercial insurance and Medicaid funding for psychological services directed at the mental health problems of children and adolescents. Access to these funds, however, almost always requires a DSM-IV classification, and the person within a school system most qualified to deal with the issue of psychiatric classification is the school psychologist.

As a clinical psychologist, I have focused on the assessment and evaluation of human behavior during most of my professional career. Based on my experience, I have no hesitation in asserting that the school psychologists I have known and worked with over the years are just as capable of making competent psychiatric classifications as their colleagues in clinical and counseling psychology. Understanding maladjustment is an essential task for all applied psychologists, and the DSM-IV classification system is an important tool in working with psychopathology. I believe that psychologists in all applied specialties need to develop and maintain a role in the ongoing development and application of this tool. To do otherwise is to risk becoming increasingly irrelevant in the field of mental health.

The application of professional psychology is a legally regulated activity in all states. State licensing laws differ in their recognition of formal psychiatric diagnosis as a role for the psychologist. Any psychologist considering expanding his or her professional role should seek appropriate training and supervision, and should also carefully review any legal regulations pertaining to this potential area of new practice (see the following Professional Note). Consultation with an

---

PROFESSIONAL NOTE   Review of District Policies and State Regulations Regarding Mental Health Diagnosis

As a school psychologist or allied mental health professional prepares to confront the practical issues of psychiatric diagnosis, it is also prudent to review relevant agency guidelines and statutory regulation of this activity. School districts, special education units, and other employers may have formal or informal policies covering the use of behavioral classification. The professional action of diagnosing a mental disorder may be regulated or licensed by the state. Reviewing relevant policy and statutes, seeking input from professional associations, and consultation with more experienced peers can all serve to highlight potential problems, identify appropriate solutions, and reduce the anxiety commonly felt when one is moving into a new area of professional development. Some state associations for school psychologists have developed recommendations for seeking third-party reimbursement that address the issue of diagnosis (see, e.g., Elliott et al., 1993).

---

attorney who has expertise in mental health practice may well be advisable in such situations. These prudent cautions notwithstanding, I am convinced that developing expertise with using the DSM-IV classification system to codify the emotional and behavioral problems of children and adolescents is an appropriate professional activity for school psychologists. Furthermore, I believe that such expertise will be increasingly called upon and that the use of DSM-IV will eventually become an essential activity of school psychologists, just as it currently is for clinical and counseling psychologists.

BEST-PRACTICE RECOMMENDATIONS FOR SCHOOL PSYCHOLOGISTS REGARDING DIAGNOSIS

No single activity alone is sufficient for the development of a new area of competence. The school psychologist wishing to develop novel skills in mental health diagnosis should proceed exactly the same way as in the development of any other new set of skills. Reading and study, continuing educational workshops, supervised practice, and frequent professional consultation throughout the early stages of independent practice are all part of the ongoing professional development of all psychologists. Providing documentation of one's preparation to engage in various aspects of professional psychology is a common expectation, and the school psychologist should do this just as carefully as he or she develops skills in mental health diagnosis. Everything from the casual inquiry of a straightforwardly curious colleague to the pointed examination of an attorney for whom a particular classification is not a welcome development can present the school psychologist with an opportunity to explain how he or she engages in mental health diagnosis and how he or she has prepared for this role.

CHAPTER 13

The Case Record:
Data and Supporting
Documentation for Diagnosis

♦

The case record of a child or adolescent contains all the essential records and documentation necessary for the provision of psychological services. Part of this record should include the mental health classification made and any relevant data bearing on the issue of diagnosis. As an intern, I was required to note after any diagnosis the data supporting this classification: for example, "Conduct Disorder as manifested by . . . ." This was a good habit to develop, and in my case notes I still make a point of listing the signs and symptoms supporting any working or final diagnoses. The best way to defend any diagnostic statement made is to point out the behavioral phenomena that form the basis for the classification. Because mental health records may follow an individual for a very long time, it is essential that sufficient documentation and data be maintained to allow a future review of any diagnosis.

CONFIDENTIALITY, FREEDOM OF INFORMATION, AND PARENTS' AND CHILDREN'S RIGHTS

An important topic to consider in the professional activity of any psychologist is maintaining the privacy and confidentiality of information about clients. In additional to the ethical requirements of the profession, there are in most states specific legal requirements governing the protection and circumstances for legal release of psychological records. If mental health classification becomes a part of a child or adolescent's school records, it is advisable to determine whether additional legal requirements regarding confidentiality apply. The statutes governing mental health information may differ from those covering educational data. Mental health confidentiality laws can be complex, especially for adolescents, who may be treated as more autonomous than children but not yet fully emancipated.

Schools are usually held responsible not only for withholding information without appropriate releases, but also for providing information to parents or other legal guardians. This typically includes mental health information. The practicing psychologist needs to be comfortable discussing a client's psychiatric diagnosis with a mature client or the parents of an immature client, or, in the case of a teenager, with both the adolescent and his or her parents. Again, it is important to be familiar with the specific legal mandates that apply a particular state, and with the policies and procedures of a particular work setting. With the issue of mental health classification, there may not be a policy in effect because such classification has not been a practice within that school system in the past. Developing a written policy may be one of the first tasks for the school psychologist who has moved into this area of practice.

It is good practice to maintain a record of any information disclosed from a case record. If the release is to be of copies of records, I routinely note on the release-of-information form what documents were copies, to whom they were transmitted, and the date. If the release is oral, I include a summary of the information discussed in my case notes.

MAINTENANCE OF RECORDS

Mental health records need to be maintained securely, both to protect clients' confidentiality and to provide for their legitimate release at the clients' request. The importance of a longitudinal data base seems undeniable in our attempts to understand human development, both adaptive and maladaptive, more clearly. The most solid basis for resolving difficult diagnostic questions is often the course a young person's problem takes over time.

Providing for the secure storage and maintenance of records should not be a new responsibility for any school system. It may, however, be prudent to review state requirements for maintenance of records with respect to mental health records, if DSM-IV diagnoses are being added to the case data generated within school records (see the following Professional Note). As I have noted above, laws may differ for mental health records versus educational records. If DSM-IV diagnoses are included in a child's psychological, file it is likely that these records will be considered mental health records by a court and that the applicable confidentiality acts will apply.

PROFESSIONAL NOTE   Maintenance of Mental Health Records

One variation of a common joke among psychologists and other mental health professionals is the following: "How long should mental health records be retained? Forever plus 7 years." Although there is no absolute answer to the question this joke poses, it is an important practical issue for both the school psychologist and the school district. The relevant state statutes governing appropriate handling of mental health records may differ from those pertaining to educational records. In addition, the potential role mental health records may play if a question of professional malpractice or liabiity is ever raised is an important consideration. The school psychologist should carefully consider the issues regarding maintenance of mental health records, and the school district should develop a formal policy (if none exists). A review of documents such as the American Psychological Association's (1993) guidelines is a good starting point.

CHAPTER 14

◆◆◆

Seeking Reimbursement
for Assessment and Diagnosis
within School Settings

◆

PHYSICIANS' CURRENT PROCEDURAL
TERMINOLOGY CODES

The *Physicians' Current Procedural Terminology* (CPT; American Medical Association, 1992) is a system used to identify medical procedures, including diagnostic procedures. It was originally developed by the American Medical Association in 1966 as a means of reporting the services performed by physicians. The CPT codes were revised in 1970, 1973, and 1977, and the 1977 (fourth) edition is updated annually (Schmidt, 1993). The CPT gives descriptive phrases to identify professional activities and assigns a five-digit code to each one (e.g., "psychological testing" is coded 96100). It provides a uniform method of documenting health care activities, and especially of communicating with third-party payers (insurance companies, state or federal government agencies). The 1983 update of CPT was adopted by the Health Care Financing Administration (HCFA) as part of that agency's common procedural coding system for reporting services to the Medicare and Medicaid programs, and subsequent revisions have continued to serve as the primary basis for accessing these potential sources of reimbursement (Schmidt, 1993). Most insurance companies require CPT codes to be used in all claims submitted. The school psychologist or school system seeking reimbursement from insurance companies or public programs will usually need to be able to document these claims in terms of these codes. Schmidt's (1993) brief "companion volume" is a good introduction to the CPT and has very useful sections on dealing with third-party carriers and documenting mental health services. Most of the professional activity involved in psychological evaluation and diagnosis is reflected in the following CPT codes: 90801 (initial diagnostic interview), 96100 (psychological testing), and 90825 (review of records) (see the following Coding Note for more codes).

Submission of claims to most third-party payers either requires or is greatly facilitated by the use of a standard health insurance claim form, usually identified as the HCFA-1500 form. This form (available from many companies providing business supplies for medical settings and physicians) provides a standardized format for the recording of information on the patient, his or her insurance, the medical procedures conducted, and their relationship to diagnoses, as well as information on the provider of the services. As with any complex system, initial experiences with the HCFA-1500 can be quite frustrating; however, the range of potential psychological services and procedures

---

CODING NOTE   Examples of CPT-4 Codes Relevant to Psychologists

90801	Initial diagnostic interview, outpatient, per hour
90825	Review of records
96100	Psychological testing with interpretation and report, per hour (formerly 90830)
96111	Developmental testing with interpretation and report, ex tended, per hour (formerly 95881)
96110	Developmental testing, limited (new code)
96117	Neuropsychological testing battery with interpretation and report, per hour (formerly 95883)
90841	Individual psychotherapy; time unspecified
90842	Individual psychotherapy; approximately 75 to 80 minutes
90843	Individual psychotherapy; approximately 20 to 30 minutes
90844	Individual psychotherapy; approximately 45 to 50 minutes
90846	Family psychotherapy (without the patient present)
90847	Family psychotherapy (conjoint psychotherapy)
90853	Group psychotherapy

CPT codes are frequently revised and updated. Prior to submitting any actual billing it is wise to check the most current codes. The insurance company will usually provide this if necessary. CPT only ©1998 American Medical Association. All Rights Reserved.

---

is really very limited, and billing for psychological evaluation can usually become the province of the technical support staff after some initial familiarity with the form has been gained. (Of course, regardless of who completes a form, the licensed psychologist who signs the form is responsible for the accuracy of the information contained and should carefully review any submission for reimbursement.)

The diagnosis item of the HCFA-1500 calls for an ICD-9-CM code. This is the numerical code that is associated with a DSM-IV diagnosis. For instance, the DSM-IV diagnosis of Oppositional Defiant Disorder has the ICD-9-CM code 313.81. All DSM-IV diagnoses are legitimate ICD-9-CM diagnoses; that is, all DSM-IV diagnoses have ICD-9-CM code numbers assigned to them. However, not every DSM-IV diagnosis has its own ICD-9-CM code. As some of the "Coding Note" figures in Part II of this book have pointed out, several DSM-IV diagnoses may have the same code number assigned to them. In addition, the 10th revision of the ICD classification system is currently being adopted for use in the United States, and ICD codes will change when this transition is complete.

"MEDICAL NECESSITY" AS A CRITERION

Commercial insurance companies and governmental insurance programs (Medicare, Medicaid, Social Security, Civilian Health and Medicaid Program of the Uniformed Services [CHAMPUS]) employ various controls and restrictions on the reimbursement for medical services. Much of the attention is focused on the reimbursement of treatment, but evaluations will also fall under these guidelines if assessment services are covered by an insurance policy. Typically, the policy will indicate that only services that are "medically necessary," or some other phrase to this effect will be considered for potential reimbursement. Some policies will only reimburse for services if a referral has been made by a physician. The final determination of what is "medically necessary" is often made by the third-party payer.

Some insurance companies, for instance, may not deem it appropriate to reimburse for psychological services to treat an adolescent with problems of isolated antisocial behavior (V71.02, Adolescent Antisocial Behavior—an "Other Conditions That May Be a Focus of Clinical Attention" classification) because this is not a mental Disorder. The same insurance company may help pay for the very same services in another young person if the diagnosis is 312.82, Conduct Disorder, Adolescent-Onset Type, or 309.3, Adjustment Disorder With

Disturbance of Conduct. These differing determinations can be frustrating for the psychologist, because the very same psychological services may be provided in both cases. The decision does make sense from the perspective of the insurance company, however. In the second case, the problem is identified as a Mental Disorder. The holder of the insurance policy has paid for coverage of mental disorders, and it is the obligation of the insurance company to provide this coverage. Note that the insurance company does not have an obligation either to provide unlimited help to the policy holder, or to support the psychologist providing the services in "doing good." The obligations of the insurer to the insured are very specifically laid out in the insurance policy. Despite frequent advertisement themes suggesting that insurance companies are policy holders' friends and will watch out for them, the actual relationship is carefully governed by contract and law. One should consider that to reimburse a claim not covered under a holder's contract would be an unethical act for the insurance company. Such behavior would reduce the legitimate profits of the shareholders of the company and could ultimately lead to rate increases for all policy holders.

With respect to determining psychiatric diagnoses, assessment and evaluation services may often be more broadly covered under a mental health policy than treatment services may be. For instance, in some cases the evaluation of a potential mental disorder may be determined to be eligible for reimbursement, even if the condition is ultimately diagnosed is one that is not eligible for coverage. As long as an eligible condition is being actively considered in the evaluation process (i.e., being "ruled out"), this process itself may be eligible. Individual policies vary widely, however, and it is never safe to rely on generalizations about psychological conditions, services, or insurance companies. What matters is the exact insurance contract that the client has purchased with the third-party carrier or the contract that has been negotiated by the client's employer.

Potential insurance reimbursement for any psychological service will depend on the exact nature of coverage for mental health services in the insured's policy. Most policies covering mental health services have "deductibles" that must be satisfied prior to recovery of any funds; will typically reimburse only a portion of "the usual and customary fees" for a service in that area; and/or may have yearly or lifetime "caps" for a particular disorder, which set an upper limit on the amount of potential total reimbursement. A good deal of unhappiness can be avoided by carefully and accurately determining how services will be paid for before these services are provided. Clients often overestimate how helpful their health insurance policies will be in supporting mental health services. Small's (1993) text is a valuable reference on this topic.

ETHICAL AND PROFESSIONAL RESPONSIBILITIES IN BILLING

School psychologists usually have a great deal of experience in carrying out psychological evaluations. The output of these evaluations may not have been expressed in the language of DSM-IV, but the process of careful and accurate assessment has been well developed in every competently trained school psychologist. Applying these skills to the use of the DSM-IV classification system is really a minor extension. School psychologists, usually by both natural inclination and formal training, also have a mental set to be helpful to their clients— to provide as much assistance as possible to young people, their teachers, and their parents and families. However, school psychologists usually have not had much experience in billing for psychological services and in interacting with insurance companies or other third-party carriers. This creates the potential for some difficulties.

School psychologists who are moving into the role of seeking reimbursement for psychological services need to think very carefully through their professional role and responsibilities. The job of a school psychologist carrying out a psychological evaluation is to make the best assessment of the young person and of his or her situation that is possible under the circumstances. The job of such a psychologist who makes use of the DSM-IV classification system is to express the results in the most appropriate DSM-IV code or codes—to choose the DSM-IV category or categories that most accurately and validly capture the essential features of this child's or adolescent's situation. The job of the school psychologist is *not* to help the school system or the young person's parents obtain insurance reimbursement for the care given in the case. At least, it is not directly the responsibility of the school psychologist to do anything and everything possible to achieve reimbursement.

Certainly the psychologist should be willing to provide records (with appropriately executed releases of information) to support insurance claims; the school system may even file the claims; and it may even be part of the psychologist's job to file the claims (not a very efficient use of professional time, though it does happen). But the issue of potential reimbursement must not enter into any decision about classification. Neither the Axis I and II diagnoses nor the Global Assessment of Functioning rating on Axis V can be influenced by what may happen when the case is reviewed by an insurance company for possible reimbursement under a medical insurance policy. Reimbursement decisions have no place in decisions about diagnosis. If these considerations are given a place in diagnostic classification, the basic validity of the process is violated. The integrity of the evaluation has been lost. To base a diagnosis on anything other than the behavioral facts of the case is unethical. If such a diagnosis is used to try to obtain reimbursement, this is usually illegal—an act of fraud against the insurance company or other third-party payer.

Graduate students in diagnostic classes are very anxious about making mistakes. They are very concerned over disagreements regarding diagnosis. They want very much to be sure that their diagnoses are correct. Although such concerns are understandable and reasonable up to a point, the reality is that each diagnosis of human behavior is at best a calculated hypothesis based on the data known at that time. Subsequently acquired information may require a change in the diagnosis. This does not mean that the first diagnosis was wrong and the second is right; both have been based on the data available. As I have repeatedly pointed out in this text, clinical judgment continues to play the decisive role in the DSM-IV classification system. Clinical judgment is the interpretation of the available data by the diagnosing professional—the weighing of various bits of information that support the diagnosis offered. A great deal of effort has gone into making the DSM-IV criteria as objective as possible, but there is still a great deal of room for honest differences of opinion. Two examiners may legitimately reach different final classifications of an individual case. Although we should strive to resolve such differences whenever possible, their occurrence cannot be eliminated from the application of DSM-IV. Neither the profession nor society at large expects perfect agreement; however, psychologists are expected to operate within the rules. The ultimate rule for proper psychiatric diagnosis is that classification needs to be based on the behavioral data available for each case. A psychologist who has proceeded on this basis will be able to show the justification for the classification. Even if it is later determined that this diagnosis is not correct, I believe that there is little risk for either the psychologist or his or her agency. Again, society does not expect psychologists to be perfect, but it does expect psychologists to operate within their own rules. If a diagnosis is based on any consideration other than the known facts of the case, then a psychologist does assume a great risk, both personally and for the public status and reputation of psychology.

DIAGNOSTIC DISAGREEMENT

A related issue concerns agreement among diagnosticians. One driving force behind the wholesale changes introduced in DSM-III, which has continued to reverberate in the subsequent revisions, was the need for better reliability in psychiatric diagnosis. As differential treatments began to become available for a number of psychiatric disorders, a need for treatment evaluation research developed. Such research, however, required a reliable and valid classification system to establish treatment and control groups. There was general recognition of the unreliability of DSM-II, and without adequate reliability, validity was a moot concern. The objectivity, explicit criterion sets, and diagnostic decision rules of DSM-III, DSM-III-R, and DSM-IV were intended to increase the reliability to an acceptable level. A review of the field study data suggests that considerable progress has been made toward this end. Given access to the same data, different evaluators are probably more likely to arrive at the same or related diagnoses with DSM-IV than with any previous classification tool.

"Given access to the same data," however, is the key phrase in the last sentence of the preceding paragraph. Mental health professionals do not always have the same information to work with. Developing skills in eliciting diagnostic data efficiently and comprehensively is a major career task for professionals from diverse disciplines. The task of obtaining the necessary data to arrive at DSM-IV diagnoses is beyond the intention or capacity of this text, but other references do address this important topic (Kronenberger & Meyer, 1996; Meyer & Deitsch, 1996; Othmer & Othmer, 1994a, 1994b). One clear advantage of DSM-IV is a relatively clear formulation of what types of information are helpful and necessary to establish, support, and document a diagnostic formulation.

The task of the evaluator is always to make the best, most accurate classification based on the specific data available for a child or adolescent at the time. It needs to be emphasized that this formulation will not always agree with previous or future assessments by different mental health professionals, or even by the same professional. If a diagnosis is based on the best formulation of all of the data that are available at that time, it is the correct diagnosis. Other professionals may have the benefit of additional historical facts, collateral reports, clinical observations, reports of responses to treatment efforts, and/or further course data. Based in part on all these data, new formulations of the young person's difficulties may be generated. This does not mean that the original diagnosis was wrong or incorrect. Again, if the diagnosis was based fairly on the known information at that time, then it was the correct diagnosis. A revision of a diagnostic formulation does not imply an error on anyone's part. Neither does a difference of opinion between two professionals involved in a child's or adolescent's care. As has been previously noted, DSM-IV provides substantial opportunities for clinical judgment, differential evaluation of the functional significance of symptomatic behavior, and attention to idiosyncratic features of a case to influence case formulations. However, this flexibility comes at a cost: Different mental health professionals will not always see a young person's case as best formulated in the same way. The DSM system does provide a framework that can be used for an objective review of diagnostic differences, but these will not always be completely resolved.

To reiterate once more, the school psychologist's job is to evaluate a child's or adolescent's emotional and behavioral problems in a fair, objective, and comprehensive manner, and to base his or her diagnostic formulation on the facts that are currently available—not on concerns about reimbursement or on any other considerations. If another professional arrives at a different diagnosis, this is interesting, but it does not necessarily have any implications for the psychologist's work. All professionals need to be willing to consider new information as it becomes available. A diagnosis may be revised in the light of new data, but this does not mean that the previous classification was in error. It may have been completely accurate based on the understanding then available of the young person and his or her situation.

CHAPTER 15

DSM-IV and the Individuals with Disabilities Education Act

◆

Specific comparisons between the classifications of DSM-IV and those of the Individuals with Disabilities Education Act of 1990 (IDEA; P.L. 101-476) have been made in the IDEA Notes throughout Part II of this text. From a more general perspective, I believe that the most important consideration for the school psychologist or other child care professional is to recognize that, despite clear commonalities, the DSM-IV and IDEA systems constitute two very different perspectives on children's adjustment problems. DSM-IV and IDEA both classify patterns of behavior shown by children and are both categorical in their approach to classification. Both have a primary application in the allocation of resources (special services, treatments, medications, placement dispositions) for children. Both are carefully constructed human documents, in which classifications have been arrived at through consideration of divergent viewpoints, empirical data, debate, and compromise. However, beyond these important similarities are major differences in coverage, focus, methodology, and purpose, which result in two qualitatively different taxonomies of behavior. In my opinion, direct translation between DSM-IV and IDEA is not possible. The diagnostic categories of DSM-IV do not usually "map onto" any simple set or subset of IDEA categories, even when there are major overlaps of clinical elements (e.g., autism, learning disability, and mental retardation).

The coverage of DSM-IV is very broad by intention; it attempts to classify all significant problems of behavior and adjustment. Some critics of the significant conceptual and methodological changes that occurred with DSM-III raised concern that the DSM system had become too inclusive—that issues of life adjustment and minor problems of common human experience had been recast as "mental disorders" to expand the domain of psychiatry or medicine. Even if this concern is set aside, everyone would agree that the intended coverage of DSM-IV is vastly greater than the range focused upon by IDEA. A number of the mental disorders of DSM-IV are irrelevant for the purposes of IDEA. DSM-IV focuses on identifying problematic patterns of behavior that cause great personal suffering or obvious impairment in life adaptation (mental disorders) or are judged to be appropriate objects of therapeutic treatment or other intervention (V codes). By contrast, IDEA focuses on identifying psychological or medical disabilities that would prevent a child or adolescent in benefiting fairly from a public education unless appropriate remediation is made. It appears to me that many (but not all) DSM-IV mental disorders and some V codes affecting children and adolescents fall within the conceptualization of disability under IDEA; however, the correspondence is not perfect and often depends on features others than a diagnosis per se (e.g., the particular manifestations of the mental disorder or condition, the settings affected, and the impact on global adjustment).

The methodology of DSM-IV establishes objective criteria for the documentation of a Mental Disorder, but, with a few important exceptions, the methods of obtaining data relevant to these symptomatic criteria are left up to the examiner. The role of clinical judgment is extremely important, as is consistent with the origins of DSM-IV within the discipline of clinical medicine. The exact criteria used for the categories of IDEA are left to an important degree up to individual states and even to individual school districts. The methods of data collection, analysis, and determination of data quality and acceptability, however, are spelled out in IDEA and its revisions: nondiscriminatory and multidisciplinary assessment, parental involvement, and individualized educational plans. These important functional differences derive from the different purposes of these two efforts. DSM-IV is ultimately aimed at reliable and valid classification for the purposes of clinical treatment and research to improve clinical treatment. IDEA is ultimately aimed at providing safeguards so that all U.S. children have a fair and equal opportunity to benefit from public education. These are both important and laudable goals, but they are different; thus, the products of these two efforts are different, even when they sound alike (e.g., "mental retardation" in IDEA and Mental Retardation in DSM-IV).

The definition of "behavioral disorders" offered within the IDEA legislation has itself been criticized on a number of grounds (Cline, 1990; Council for Children with Behavioral Disorders, 1987; Forness & Knitzer, 1990), and alternative definitions have been proposed (Forness & Knitzer, 1990). Even within the federal government, there is incongruity between different definitions of "serious emotional disturbance" (Substance Abuse and Mental Health Services Administration, 1993). This will be a subject of continuing discussion and debate as the United States struggles to accommodate the various educational, economic, political, medical, social, and psychological needs and realities that affect child learning and development. Documentation of a DSM-IV mental disorder will often, perhaps usually, have relevance for a potential classification of a child or adolescent as eligible for special education or other special services under IDEA. The information involved in a DSM-IV diagnosis (symptoms, severity, course, effects, prognosis) will almost always be relevant, either positively or negatively, to establishment of eligibility under IDEA. Yet the categories of DSM-IV are not identical to those of IDEA. Some of the differences are perhaps minor differences in boundaries (e.g., age or degree of mental retardation), in formulations (the molar categories of IDEA vs. the molecular categories of DSM-IV), or in exact labels. The fundamental reality, however, is that some children with a DSM-IV diagnosis of a mental disorder are not as eligible for services under IDEA, and that some children who are eligible for services under IDEA do not have a mental disorder as defined by DSM-IV. These are related but separate classification questions. The school psychologist may play a vital role in each determination, but each type of inquiry asks a unique question and deserves its own unique answer.

CHAPTER 16

♦♦♦

Concerns about DSM-IV

♦

This text has not addressed the various pros and cons of psychiatric classification. These have been argued repeatedly, and there is good reason to continue considering the issue. No one who has walked the halls of a school for any length of time can really question the assertion that words can hurt. Labels (informal or formal) can be hurled as weapons, and the emotional pain that can result is just as palpable as physical pain. The possibility of an accidental disclosure of a young person's mental health diagnosis, and the ensuing potential for mischief and peer cruelty, are very real concerns. But words can also provide relief and a better understanding. Sometimes just having a name for a problem, as well as understanding that other young people have gone though similar difficulties, can provide comfort and the beginnings of self-acceptance. I view psychiatric classification as a tool to be used in helping to deal with human problems. Like all tools, it can be used well or badly, and can have good or bad effects on people's lives. We need the best tools available, and we need to use these tools well. A deficiency in either the quality of our instruments or our application of them can decrease our effectiveness.

The strengths and weaknesses of DSM-IV as a classification system in general, and the use of DSM-IV with children in particular, have received a good deal of critical attention. This is as it should be; vigorous evaluation can only benefit future attempts to portray the challenges of human adjustment more usefully. In the present text, I have assumed that a decision to use DSM-IV has already been made, and have paid little attention to the various conceptual, empirical, and practical criticisms of using DSM-IV with adults or children. Before closing, however, I wish to touch at least briefly on some of the major concerns that have been advanced by various investigators and practitioners. For fuller treatment of this important area, and citations of the growing literature of critical analysis, the reader is referred to Achenbach and McConaughy (1996), Jensen and Hoagwood (1997), and Scotti, Morris, McNeil, and Hawkins (1996).

CONCERNS ABOUT PSYCHIATRIC CLASSIFICATION IN GENERAL

The concerns that have been expressed about the use of DSM-IV often begin with reservations about psychiatric diagnosis in general children and then go on to the specific real or potential weaknesses of this particular system of classification. The general concerns frequently discussed include issues of inviting bias and stigmatization, unfairly portraying clients as somehow responsible for their behavior problems ("blaming the victims"), contributing to a false and premature closure of inquiry as a client is assigned a diagnosis, oversimplifying complex human problems, and ignoring important individual differences. These concerns can be voiced about any systematic classification of abnormal behavior. Potential alternative solutions include not classifying behavior at all (if this is possible), using purely idiographic or functional analyses of behavior, or identifying behavior change needs in more positive terms (idealistic or growth-based conceptualizations of behavior). DSM-IV may be used as a specific example of the problems inherent in psychiatric classification, but the concerns are often not limited to this system. It is the endeavor of classifying human problems itself that is seen as fraught with negative consequences for those we wish to assist.

In one sense these discussions are truly "academic," because we do classify people both formally and informally, and will continue do so as long as there are differential assignments, treatments, learning environments, and resources to allocate. In a more fundamental sense, however, such debates are very important: These concerns and exchanges serve to remind us to consider the effects of our actions. There is a link, unfortunately, between the clinical diagnosis of Mental Retardation in a child's chart and the painful taunt of "Retard!" hurled across the playground. Though I believe that we cannot eliminate the insults by banning the diagnoses, it would be foolish to ignore the reality that our words can have many unintended consequences. Substituting new labels is only a very temporary solution. A few years ago, "developmental disability" began to become the preferred phrase for children with Mental Retardation. Within only a couple of months of reading the phrase used in this way in a professional journal, I heard on a local playground the epithet: "You DD!" It behooves us to consider our language on a regular basis, and to avoid terms and phrases that have taken on prejudicial or emotionally hurtful meanings; however, real progress here requires an ongoing and honest dialogue in the society at large about behavioral differences and ways to address these challenges. DSM-IV, to the degree that it is a more objective and empirically validated system of psychiatric classification than the alternatives, provides as good a foundation upon which to base this dialogue as any other.

Another significant concern is the possibility of racial or ethnic bias in psychiatric classification. Although the development of more objective diagnostic criteria almost certainly helped in this area, there was also compelling empirical evidence that problems remained in previous editions of DSM (Pavkov, Lewis, & Lyons, 1989). The authors of DSM-IV have attempted to make it more sensitive to cultural issues than any previous classification system. For example, an appendix is included in DSM-IV (Appendix I) that gives an outline for cultural formulation of a case, and provides a glossary of the most commonly discussed culture-bound syndromes in anthropology and cultural psychiatry. The *DSM-IV Casebook* (Spitzer, Gibbons, Skodol, Williams, & First, 1994) covers a number of international cases intended to increase awareness of cultural phenomena in the expression of emotional and behavioral disturbances.

Despite these efforts, many fundamental questions remain about the best ways to understand cultural differences in efforts to classify adjustment problems (Stein, 1993). Cervantes and Arroyo (1994) have discussed the use of DSM-IV with Hispanic children and adolescents, and make a number of recommendations aimed at minimizing potential cultural biases in applying the classification system to this expanding segment of the population. As Cervantes and Arroyo point out, there are currently few empirical data to work with in this area, but publications such as theirs can provide a good impetus for research and for public discussion. Both empirical study and open dialogue are need to promote culturally appropriate services for minorities.

Novins and colleagues (1997) have recently presented an illustration of the DSM-IV approach with Native American children. They discuss both DSM-IV's improved coverage and its continuing limitations with respect to ethnicity and cultural background. There are no absolute guidelines to apply to these questions. Even the idea of "culture-bound syndromes" has been questioned by some (Bartholomew, 1995). Yet few would debate the assertion that our cultural heritage affects behavior, and therefore aberrations of that behavior, in a pervasive way. Psychologists have begun to develop greater sensitivity for how culture and ethnic background can affect psychological testing (Cervantes & Acosta, 1992; Dauphinais & King, 1992), and DSM-IV has advanced this perspective into diagnostic formulations. Although many questions, concerns, and challenges remain, it is at the very least a good beginning.

CONCERNS ABOUT DSM-IV'S OVERALL CONCEPTUALIZATION AND STRUCTURE

On a still general level, but pertaining more directly to DSM-IV, are concerns about the overall conceptualization and structure of this taxonomic system. DSM-IV uses a categorical model, relies on clinical assessment, allows multiple diagnoses, and often employs polycritic (in which, say, 3 of a list of 7 symptoms are enough to satisfy a criterion) criterion sets. These features have all received both positive and negative comment.

Levy, Hay, McStephen, Wood, and Waldman (1997) analyzed data from a cohort of 1,938 families and concluded that Attention-Deficit/Hyperactivity Disorder (ADHD) is best viewed as an extreme expression of behavior that varies along a continuum, rather than as a categorical disorder. Shaywitz, Escobar, et al. (1990) have raised similar concerns about "dyslexia." Questions have also been asked about depression, anxiety, substance use, social isolation, autistic thinking, reality testing, eating disturbances, sleep problems, and virtually every other difficulty formulated within DSM-IV. Yet even when human variability may be continuous, our responses to it are not. A child either goes to the reading resource room during third period or does not, a prescription for a stimulant medication is made or not; counseling sessions are recommended or not. As long as specific dispositions are to be made, then even a continuous variable will be dichotomized in some manner: Up to a certain point, a young person continues with regular classes; if the variable is more extreme than this, an alternative plan is put in motion.

The ultimate reliance on clinical judgment and decision making in the DSM-IV system has been commented upon several times already. It is both a strength and a weakness of DSM-IV. Human judgment and decision making, guided by clear statements and objective criteria, offer the most sophisticated and subtle problem-solving solutions possible. The human mind is capable of weighing multiple factors to arrive at a conclusion; at the present time, no mechanical decision-making algorithm is superior to it over the range of activity covered in DSM-IV. At the same time, this reliance on clinical judgment brings with it possibilities of bias, idiosyncratic decisions, errors, and intentional circumventions of the diagnostic criteria. Individual evaluators are responsible for the quality and accuracy of their diagnostic assignments. Ongoing education, consultation, and review of previous decisions are essential for the appropriate and accurate application of DSM-IV.

Another body of misgivings about DSM-IV relates to the number of diagnostic categories and the frequent occurrence of multiple diagnoses. The system has been criticized as too complicated, with too many diagnoses that a practitioner will not reliably make discriminations between. The usual observation that comorbidity of psychiatric diagnoses is the rule rather than the exception with DSM-IV also causes concern. The ICD system, through most of its editions, has sought to reduce the number of behavioral classifications by an emphasis on making a single mental health diagnosis and by the use of combined categories (e.g., "mixed anxiety and depressive disorder"). The deliberate strategy of providing a wide array of behavioral classifications and of allowing concurrent diagnoses speaks to the intention of DSM-IV's authors to provide the most comprehensive accounting of mental health problems possible. The basic reality is that human behavior is fantastically complex and problematic manifestations are no less so, and most of us have not isolated difficulties but combinations of problems. DSM-IV attempts to mirror as fully as possible the range and nature of human behavioral problems. In doing so, it necessarily takes on a complex and elaborate form. Efforts to hold down or reduce the number of categories proceed hand in hand with efforts to achieve even finer degrees of differentiation (and hence more categories and probably more multiple categorizations).

SPECIFIC CONCERNS ABOUT DSM-IV

On yet another level are specific concerns or criticisms regarding the axes, categories, criteria, and diagnostic thresholds of DSM-IV—both those carried over from DSM-III-R, and the new formulations being used and evaluated for the first time.

The relationship between classifications of behavior problems in children versus adolescents versus adults remains a continuing concern. Several of the "child" diagnoses in DSM-III-R have been absorbed into the thematic areas of diagnosis (Mood Disorders, Anxiety Disorders, etc.) in DSM-IV. Greater attention has also been given to identifying developmentally characteristic symptom manifestations within several criterion sets (e.g., Posttraumatic Stress Disorder in children and ADHD in adults). Continued epidemiological and general population studies continue to increase our understanding of the typical onset and course of autism, attention problems, and mood disturbances, to name only a few. Despite these efforts, the most useful boundaries and conceptualizations to capture the difficulties of childhood and adolescence remain subjects of much contention and debate. For example, a significant amount of effort went into the multisite field trials of proposed Disruptive Behavior Disorder categories for DSM-IV. In spite of this effort, there remains a great deal of dissatisfaction over the boundaries between categories (e.g., Conduct Disorder and Oppositional Defiant Disorder) and within categories (e.g., the Predominantly Inattentive and Predominantly Hyperactive–Impulsive Types of ADHD).

Empirical studies of a number of diagnostic categories have concluded with remarkably consistent findings: (1) Diagnostic threshold translates directly into the size of the population identified as showing a given problem; (2) a more inclusive definition increases the heterogeneity of, and reduces the average severity of disturbance in, the population identified; and (3) in the usual absence of a "gold standard" of diagnostic correctness, there is not usually a natural break clearly demonstrating the superiority of one threshold of symptom frequency over another. As increasingly differentiated intervention and therapy options become available, the potential costs of false-positive versus false-negative errors may play an increasing role in future formulations of diagnostic systems. The challenge of differential diagnosis will remain an area of ongoing concern over the life of DSM-IV, and various tools and approaches to address this need will continue to appear (e.g., First et al., 1995).

The greater emphasis on clinically significant impairment incorporated into most of the diagnostic categories of DSM-IV pertaining to children and adolescents also deserves some comment. The understandable intent was to decrease false-positive diagnoses of minor or trivial problems of life as mental disorders because particular patterns of very mild intensity happened to meet the "formal" diagnostic criteria. The purpose of DSM-IV's definition of mental disorders is clearly to identify and classify abnormal patterns of action and feelings. This emphasis also leads to a greater focus on Axis V, the Global Assessment of Functioning (GAF) rating. The GAF rating of all mental disorders presumably reflects their defined nature; one would usually expect GAF ratings below 70 for any fully manifested mental disorder. Fundamental questions regarding the application of Axis V remain unanswered, however. How reliable are DSM-IV Axis V rat-

ings across different professionals, over time, and for different diagnostic categories? How sensitive are Axis V ratings to the natural course
of a disorder and to therapeutic response? How valid are the ratings
as indices of real-life adjustment, school performance, social functioning, and vocational success? Empirical data on DSM-IV GAF ratings are lacking, but the scale is essentially identical to Axis V in DSM-
III and DSM-III-R. The available data on previous versions of the GAF
scale raise concerns about its reliability across evaluators (van Goor-
Lambo, 1987). Research and development to learn the best ways to
train examiners in the use of Axis V and to maintain reliability of
their GAF ratings is greatly needed.

The extent of, and dependence upon various methodologies of,
data collection constitute another area of continued questions regarding DSM-IV. As noted earlier in this book, DSM-IV calls for formal
psychological or other assessment for only a few diagnostic decisions
(Mental Retardation, Learning Disorders, Communication Disorders,
certain cognitive problems). In common clinical practice, self-report
instruments, behavior rating scales, and structured interviews are frequently employed in the assessment of a variety of other problem
areas. Many investigators and practitioners working with ADHD would
insist on the use of age- and gender-normed behavior ratings of core
symptoms by one or more informants familiar with a child's behavior
in natural life settings. Self-report symptom scales are being increasingly used in the evaluation of childhood and adolescent depression,
anxiety, dissociative symptoms, and conduct problems. Both comprehensive and domain-specific structured interviews have been developed for childhood behavior problems. All of these generally positive developments bring in their own sets of methodological issues
and problems. For example, how many adult informants should complete an ADHD rating scale for a child, which scale should be used,
and how should discrepancies among reports be dealt with? The questions are multiple, important, and often without clear and definitive
answers. Auxiliary tools clearly have the potential to increase the objectivity and reliability of DSM-IV classification; realizing this potential, however, will require a great deal of empirical investigation. The
availability of objective, reliable, and empirically validated diagnostic
categories can only facilitate this ongoing, important work.

CONCLUDING REMARKS

It is my belief that the careful assessment of behavior and problems
of behavior has contributed in a basic way to our growing understand-

ing of adjustment and of psychopathology. As a part of this process, psychiatric classification has played and appears likely to continue to play an important role in research on behavioral and emotional problems of children and adolescents. Psychiatric classification also plays a significant procedural role in clinical activity; choices of medical, psychological, and educational interventions are increasingly being made on the basis of such classification. Although the DSM-IV system is not the only basis upon which evaluation can be conducted, and although (as this chapter has noted) it is by no means a perfect system, it is an important one. As the profession of psychology prepares to move into the next millennium, I believe that psychologists practicing within educational settings will see an increasing application of the DSM classification system. In their recent discussion of teacher assessments of behavioral disorders, Horwitz, Bility, Plichta, Leaf, and Haynes (1998, p. 117) point out that 12% of all children under 18 years of age have a diagnosed mental disorder—an estimated 7.5 million children and adolescents. This is a tremendous population in need of services. I believe that the professional training of psychologists provides them with a good basis upon which to practice mental health classification, and I see this activity as a professional responsibility they will increasingly be called upon to perform. I hope this text proves to be of assistance to school psychologists and other child clinical professionals who are beginning to function in this additional role.

References

♦

Abikoff, H., & Klein, R. G. (1992). Attention-deficit Hyperactivity and Conduct Disorder: *Comorbidity and implications for treatment. Journal of Consulting and Clinical Psychology, 60,* 881–892.

Achenbach, T. M., & McConaughy, S. H. (1996). Relations between DSM-IV and empirically based assessment. *School Psychology Review, 25,* 329–341.

Adams, G. B., Waas, G. A., March, J. S., & Smith, M. C. (1994). Obsessive Compulsive Disorder in children and adolescents: The role of the school psychologist in identification, assessment, and treatment. *School Psychology Quarterly, 9,* 274–294.

Aman, M. G., Hammer, D., & Rojahn, J. (1993). Mental Retardation. In T. H. Ollendick & M. Hersen (Eds.), *Handbook of child and adolescent assessment.* Needham Heights, MA: Allyn & Bacon.

Aman, M. G., Pejeau, C., Osborne, P., Rojahn, J., & Handen, B. (1996). Four-year follow-up of children with low intelligence and ADHD. *Research in Developmental Disabilities, 17,* 417–432.

American Association on Mental Retardation (AAMR). (1992). *Mental Retardation: Definition, classification, and systems of supports* (4th ed.). Washington, DC: Author.

American Medical Association. (1992). *Physicians' current procedural terminology* (4th ed.). Chicago: Author. (*Note*: Updates to this edition are published annually.)

American Psychiatric Association. (1968). *Diagnostic and statistical manual of mental disorders* (2nd ed.). Washington, DC: Author.

American Psychiatric Association (1980). *Diagnostic and statistical manual of mental misorders* (3rd ed.). Washington, DC: Author.

American Psychiatric Association. (1987). *Diagnostic and statistical manual of mental disorders* (3rd ed. rev.). Washington, DC: Author.

American Psychiatric Association. (1994a). *Diagnostic and statistical manual of mental disorders* (4th ed.). Washington, DC: Author.

American Psychiatric Association. (1994b). *Quick reference to the diagnostic criteria from DSM-IV.* Washington, DC: Author.

American Psychiatric Association. (1996a). *Coding changes to DSM-IV classification.* Washington, DC: Author.

American Psychiatric Association. (1996b). *DSM-IV coding update*. Washington, DC: Author.

American Psychiatric Association. (2000). *Diagnostic and statistical manual of mental disorders* (4th ed., text rev.). Washington, DC: Author.

American Psychological Association. (1993). Record keeping guidelines. *American Psychologist, 48,* 984–986.

American Sleep Disorders Association. (1990). *The international classification of sleep disorders: Diagnostic and coding manual*. Rochester, MN: Author.

American Sleep Disorders Association. (1997). *The international classification of sleep disorders, revised*. Rochester, MN: Author.

Angold, A., & Costello, E. J. (1996). Toward establishing an empirical basis for the diagnosis of Oppositional Defiant Disorder. *Journal of the American Academy of Child and Adolescent Psychiatry, 35,* 1205–1212.

Anthony, J. C., Warner, L. A., & Kessler, R. C. (1994). Comparative epidemiology of dependence on tobacco, alcohol, controlled substances, and inhalants: Basic findings from the National Comorbidity Survey. *Experimental and Clinical Psychopharmacology, 2,* 244–268.

Applegate, B., Lahey, B. B., Hart, E. L., Biederman, J., Hynd, G. W., Barkley, R. A., Ollendick, T., Frick, P. J., Greenhill, L., McBurnett, K., Newcorn, J. H., Kerdyk, L., Garfinkel, B., Waldman, I., & Shaffer, D. (1997). Validity of the age-of-onset criterion for ADHD: A report from the DSM-IV field trials. *Journal of the American Academy of Child and Adolescent Psychiatry, 36,* 1211–1221.

Armstrong, J. G., Putnam, F. W., Carlson, E. B., Libero, D. Z., & Smith, S. R. (1997). Development and validation of a measure of adolescent dissociation: The Adolescent Dissociative Experiences Scale. *Journal of Nervous and Mental Disease, 185,* 491–497.

Asarnow, J. R. (1994). Annotation: Childhood-onset schizophrenia. *Journal of Child Psychiatry and Psychology, 35,* 1345–1371.

Atkins, M. S., McKay, M. M., Talbott, E., & Arvanitis, P. (1996). DSM-IV diagnosis of Conduct Disorder and Oppositional Defiant Disorder: Implications and guidelines for school mental health teams. *School Psychology Review, 25,* 274–283.

August, G. J., & Garfinkel, B. D. (1989). Behavioral and cognitive subtypes of ADHD. *Journal of the American Academy of Child and Adolescent Psychiatry, 28,* 739–748.

Barkley, R. A. (1990). *Attention-deficit Hyperactivity Disorder: A handbook for diagnosis and treatment*. New York: Guilford Press.

Barkley, R. A. (1991a). Attention-deficit Hyperactivity Disorder. *Psychiatric Annals, 21,* 725–733.

Barkley, R. A. (1991b). Diagnosis and assessment of Attention-deficit Hyperactivity Disorder. *Comprehensive Mental Health Care, 1,* 27–43.

Barkley, R. A., & Biederman, J. (1997). Toward a broader definition of the age-of-onset criterion for Attention-Deficit Hyperactivity Disorder. *Journal of the American Academy of Child and Adolescent Psychiatry, 36,* 1204–1210.

Bartholomew, R. E. (1995). Culture-bound syndromes as fakery. *Skeptical Inquirer, 19,* 36–41.

Baumgaertel, A., Wolraich, M. L., & Dietrich, M. (1995). Comparison of diagnostic criteria for attention deficit disorders in a German elementary school sample. *Journal of the American Academy of Child and Adolescent Psychiatry, 34,* 629–638.

Beck, A. T., Freeman, A., & Associates (1990). *Cognitive therapy of Personality Disorders.* New York: Guilford Press.

Begali, V. (1992). *Head injury in children and adolescents: A resource and review for school and allied professionals.* Brandon, VT: Clinical Psychology.

Berman, A. L., & Schwartz, R. H. (1990). Suicide attempts among adolescent drug users. *American Journal of Diseases of Children, 144,* 310–314.

Bernstein, D. P., Cohen, P., Velez, C. N., Schwab-Stone, M., Siever, L. J., & Shinsato, L. (1993). Prevalence and stability of the DSM-III-R Personality Disorders in a community-based survey of adolescents. *American Journal of Psychiatry, 150,* 1237–1243.

Bernstein, G. A., & Borchardt, C. M. (1991). Anxiety Disorders of childhood and adolescence: A critical review. *Journal of the American Academy of Child and Adolescent Psychiatry, 30,* 519–532.

Biederman, J. (1991). Attention-deficit Hyperactivity Disorder (ADHD). *Annals of Clinical Psychiatry, 3,* 9–22.

Biederman, J. (1997). Is there a childhood form of Bipolar Disorder? *Harvard Mental Health Letter, 13,* 8.

Biederman, J., Faraone, S. V., Marrs, A., Moore, P., Garcia, J., Ablon, S., Mick, E., Gershon, J., & Kearns, M. E. (1997). Panic Disorder and Agoraphobia in consecutively referred children and adolescents. *Journal of the American Academy of Child and Adolescent Psychiatry, 36,* 214–223.

Biederman, J., Faraone, S. V., Milberger, S., Jetton, J. G., Chen, L., Mick, E., Greene, R. W., & Russell, R. L. (1996). Is childhood Oppositional Defiant Disorder a precursor to adolescent Conduct Disorder?: Findings from a four-year follow-up study of children with ADHD. *Journal of the American Academy of Child and Adolescent Psychiatry, 35,* 1193–1204.

Birmaher, B., Khetarpal, S., Brent, D., Cully, M., Balach, L., Kaufman, J., & Neer, S. M. K. (1997). The Screen for Child Anxiety Related Emotional Disorders (SCARED): Scale construction and psychometric characteristics. *Journal of the American Academy of Child and Adolescent Psychiatry, 36,* 545–553.

Birmaher, B., Ryan, N. D., Williamson, D. E., Brent, D. A., Kaufman, J., Dahl, R. E., Perel, J., & Nelson, B. (1996). Childhood and adolescent depression: A review of the past 10 years. Part I. *Journal of the American Academy of Child and Adolescent Psychiatry, 35,* 1427–1439.

Bleiberg, E. (1994). Borderline disorders in children and adolescents: The concept, the diagnosis, and the controversies. *Bulletin of the Menninger Clinic, 58,* 169–196.

Boris, N. W., Zeanah, C. H., Larrieu, J. A., Scheeringa, M. S., & Heller, S. S. (1998). Attachment disorders in infancy and early childhood: A preliminary investigation of diagnostic criteria. *American Journal of Psychiatry, 155,* 295–297.

Bradley, S. J., & Zucker, K. J. (1997). Gender Identity Disorder: A review of the past 10 years. *Journal of the American Academy of Child and Adolescent Psychiatry, 36,* 872–880.

Bregman, J. D. (1991). Current developments in the understanding of Mental Retardation: Part II. *Psychopathology. Journal of the American Academy of Child and Adolescent Psychiatry, 30,* 861–872.

Brown, G., Chadwick, O., Shaffer, D., Rutter, M., & Traub, M. (1981). A prospective study of children with head injuries: III. Psychiatric sequelae. *Psychological Medicine, 11,* 63–78.

Bryant-Waugh, R., & Lask, B. (1995). Annotation: Eating Disorders in children. *Journal of Child Psychiatry and Psychology, 36,* 191–202.

Burns, G. L., Walsh, J. A., Owens, S. M., & Snell, J. (1997). Internal validity of Attention-Deficit Hyperactivity Disorder, Oppositional Defiant Disorder, and overt Conduct Disorder symptoms in young children: Implications from teacher ratings for a dimensional approach to symptom validity. *Journal of Clinical Child Psychology, 26,* 266–275.

Campbell, M., & Malone, R. P. (1991). Mental Retardation and psychiatric disorders. *Hospital and Community Psychiatry, 42,* 374–379.

Cantwell, D., & Baker, L. (1987). *Developmental speech and language disorders.* New York: Guilford Press.

Cantwell, D., Lewinsohn, P. M., Rohde, P., & Seeley, J. R. (1997). Correspondence between adolescent report and parent report of psychiatric diagnostic date. *Journal of the American Academcy of Child and Adolescent Psychiatry, 36,* 610–619.

Carney, J., & Schoenbrodt, L. (1994). Educational implications of traumatic brain injury. *Pediatric Annals, 23,* 47–52.

Carpenter, W. T., Heinrichs, D. W., & Wagman, A. M. I. (1988). Deficit and nondeficit forms of Schizophrenia: The concept. *American Journal of Psychiatry, 145,* 578–583.

Carson, R. (1996). Aristotle, Galileo, and the DSM taxonomy: The case of Schizophrenia. *Journal of Consulting and Clinical Psychology, 64,* 1133–1139.

Centers for Disease Control and Prevention. (1996). State-specific rates of Mental Retardation—United States, 1993. *Morbidity and Mortality Weekly Report, 45,* 61–65.

Cervantes, R. C., & Acosta, F. X. (1992). Psychological testing for Hispanic Americans. *Applied and Preventive Psychology, 1,* 209–219.

Cervantes, R. C., & Arroyo, W. (1994). DSM-IV: Implications for Hispanic children and adolescents. *Hispanic Journal of Behavioral Sciences, 16,* 8–27.

Christian, R. E., Frick, P. J., Hill, N. L., Tyler, L., & Frazer, D. R. (1997). Psychopathy and conduct problems in children: II. Implications for subtyping children with conduct problems. *Journal of the American Academy of Child and Adolescent Psychiatry, 36,* 233–241.

Clarizio, H. F., & Payette, K. (1990). A survey of school psychologists' perspectives and practices with childhood depression. *Psychology in the Schools, 27,* 57–63.

Cline, D. H. (1990). A legal analysis of policy initiatives to exclude handicapped/disruptive students from special education. *Behavioral Disorders, 15,* 159–173.

Cohen-Kettenis, P. T., & van Goozen, S. H. M. (1997). Sex reassignment of adolescent transsexuals: A follow-up study. *Journal of the American Academy of Child and Adolescent Psychiatry, 36,* 263–271.

Coplan, J., & Gleason, J. R. (1988). Unclear speech: Recognition and significance of unintelligible speech in preschool children. *Pediatrics, 82,* 447–452.

Council for Children with Behavioral Disorders. (1987). Position paper on definition and identification of students with behavioral disorders. *Behavioral Disorders, 13,* 9–19.

Creak, E. M. (1961). Schizophrenic syndrome in children: Progress of a working party. *Cerebral Palsy Bulletin, 3,* 501–503.

Creak, E. M. (1963). Childhood psychosis. *British Journal of Psychiatry, 109,* 84–89.

Dauphinais, P., & King, J. (1992). Psychological assessment with American Indian children. *Applied and Preventive Psychology, 1,* 97–110.

Davila, R. R., Williams, M. L., & MacDonald, J. T. (1991, September 16). *Clarification of policy to address the needs of children with attention deficit disorders within general and/or special education.* Memorandum, U.S. Department of Education, Office of Special Education and Rehabilitative Services.

Deykin, E. Y., & Buka, S. L. (1997). Prevalence and risk factors for Posttraumatic Stress Disorder among chemically dependent adolescents. *American Journal of Psychiatry, 154,* 752–757.

Doll, B. (1996). Prevalence of psychiatric disorders in children and youth: An agenda for advocacy by school psychology. *School Psychology Quarterly, 11,* 20–47.

Dummit, E. S., III, Klein, R. G., Tancer, N. K., Asche, B., Martin, J., & Fairbanks, J. A. (1997). Systematic assessment of 50 children with Selective Mutism. *Journal of the American Academy of Child and Adolescent Psychiatry, 36,* 653–660.

Einfeld, S. L., & Aman, M. (1995). Issues in the taxonomy of psychopathology in Mental Retardation. *Journal of Autism and Developmental Disorders, 25,* 143–167.

Elliott, C., Pruett, S., Vaal, J., Agner, J., Havey, M., Boyd, L., Gallagher, R., Swerdlik, M., Berthold, M., & Lowe, J. (1993). *Best Practices for Third Party Reimbursement.* Bloomingdale, IL: Illinois School Psychologists Association (ISPA).

Emslie, G. J., Kennard, B. D., & Kowatch, R. A. (1995). Affective disorders in children: Diagnosis and management. *Journal of Child Neurology, 10*(Suppl. 1), S42–S49.

Erk, R. R. (1995). The evolution of attention deficit disorders terminology. *Elementary School Guidance and Counseling, 29,* 243–248.

Ewing-Cobbs, L., Levin, H. S., Eisenberg, H. M., & Fletcher, J. M. (1987). Language function following closed head injury in children and adolescents. *Journal of Clinical and Experimental Neuropsychology, 9*, 575–592.

Ewing-Cobbs, L., Miner, M. E., Fletcher, J. M., & Levin, H. S. (1989). Intellectual, motor, and language sequelae following closed head injury in infants and preschoolers. *Journal of Pediatric Psychology, 14*, 531–547.

Faraone, S. V., Biederman, J., Mennin, D., Wozniak, J., & Spencer, T. (1997). Attention-Deficit Hyperactivity Disorder with Bipolar Disorder: A familial subtype? *Journal of the American Academy of Child and Adolescent Psychiatry, 36*, 1378–1387.

Fay, G. C., Jaffe, K. M., Polissar, N. L., Liao, S., Rivara, J. B., & Martin, K. M. (1994). Outcome of pediatric traumatic brain injury at three years: A cohort study. *Archives of Physical Medicine and Rehabilitation, 75*, 733–741.

Federman, E. B., Costello, E. J., Angold, A., Farmer, E. M. Z., & Erkanli, A. (1997). Development of Substance Abuse and psychiatric comorbidity in an epidemiologic study of white and American Indian young adolescents: The Great Smoky Mountains Study. *Drug and Alcohol Dependence, 44*, 69–78.

First, M. B., Frances, A., & Pincus, H. A. (1995). *DSM-IV handbook of differential diagnosis.* Washington, DC: American Psychiatric Press.

Fisher, S. (1994). Identifying video game addiction in children and adolescents. *Addictive Behaviors, 19*, 545–553.

Fletcher, J. M., Ewing-Cobbs, L., Miner, M. E., Levin, H. S., & Eisenberg, H. M. (1990). Behavioral changes after closed head injury in children. *Journal of Consulting and Clinical Psychology, 58*, 93–98.

Fletcher-Flinn, C., Elmes, H., & Strugnell, D. (1997). Visual-perceptual and phonological factors in the acquisition of literacy among children with congenital Developmental Coordination Disorder. *Developmental Medicine and Child Neurology, 39*, 158–166.

Forness, S. R., & Knitzer, J. (1990). A new proposed definition and terminology to replace "serious emotional disturbance" in Individuals with Disabilities Education Act. *School Psychology Review, 21*, 12–20.

Francis, G., Last, C. G., & Strauss, C. C. (1987). Expression of Separation Anxiety Disorder: The roles of age and gender. *Child Psychiatry and Human Development, 18*, 82–89.

Francis, G., Last, C. G., & Strauss, C. C. (1992). Avoidant Disorder and Social Phobia in children and adolescents. *Journal of the American Academy of Child and Adolescent Psychiatry, 31*, 1086–1089.

Frick, P. J., Kamphaus, R. W., Lahey, B. B., Loeber, R., Christ, M. A. G., Hart, E. L., & Tannenbaum, L. E. (1991). Academic underachievement and the Disruptive Behavior Disorders. *Journal of Consulting and Clinical Psychology, 59*, 289–294.

Frick, P. J., Lahey, B. B., Applegate, B., Kerdyck, L., Ollendick, T., Hynd, G. W., Garfinkel, B., Greenhill, L., Biederman, J., Barkley, R. A., McBurnett, K., Newcorn, J., & Waldman, I. (1994). DSM-IV field trials for the Disruptive Behavior Disorders: Symptom utility estimates. *Journal of the American Academy of Child and Adolescent Psychiatry, 33*, 529–539.

Fritz, G., Fritsch, S., & Hagino, O. (1997). Somatoform Disorders in children and adolescents: A review of the past 10 years. *Journal of the American Academy of Child and Adolescent Psychiatry, 36,* 1329–1339.

Gaub, M., & Carlson, C. L. (1997). Behavioral charcteristics of DSM-IV ADHD subtypes in a school-based population. *Journal of Abnormal Child Psychology, 25,* 103–111.

Geller, B., & Luby, J. (1997). Child and adolescent Bipolar Disorder: A review of the past 10 years. *Journal of the American Academy of Child and Adolescent Psychiatry, 36,* 1168–1176.

Geller, B., Sun, K., Zimerman, B., Luby, J., Frazier, J., & Williams, M. (1995). Complex and rapid-cycling in bipolar children and adolescents: A preliminary study. *Journal of Affective Disorders, 34,* 259–268.

Giaconia, R. M., Reinherz, H. Z., Silverman, A. B., Pakiz, B., Frost, A. K., & Cohen, E. (1995). Traumas and Posttraumatic Stress Disorder in a community population of older adolescents. *Journal of the American Academy of Child and Adolescent Psychiatry, 34,* 1369–1380.

Giedd, J. N., Swedo, S. S., Lowe, C. H., & Rosenthal, N. E. (1998). Case series: Pediatric seasonal affective disorder. A follow-up report. *Journal of the American Academy of Child and Adolescent Psychiatry, 37,* 218–220.

Glaros, A. G., & Melamed, B. G. (1992). Bruxism in children: Etiology and treatment. *Applied and Preventive Psychology, 1,* 191–199.

Goldman, H. H., Skodol, A. E., & Lave, T. R. (1992). Revising Axis V for DSM-IV: A review of measures of social functioning. *American Journal of Psychiatry, 149,* 1148–1156.

Goldman, S. J., D'Angelo, E. J., Demaso, D. R., & Mezzacappa, E. (1992). Physical and sexual abuse histories among children with Borderline Personality Disorder. *American Journal of Psychiatry, 149,* 1723–1726.

Greenbaum, P. E., Foster-Johnson, L., & Petrila, A. (1996). Co-occurring addictive and mental disorders among adolescents: Prevalence research and future directions. *American Journal of Orthopsychiatry, 66,* 52–60.

Gresham, F. M., MacMillan, D. L., & Siperstein, G. N. (1995). Critical analysis of the 1992 AAMR definition: Implications for school psychology. *School Psychology Quarterly, 10,* 1–19.

Grilo, C. M., Walker, M. L., Becker, D. F., Edell, W. S., & McGlashan, T. H. (1997). Personality Disorders in adolescents with Major Depression, Substance Use Disorders, and coexisting Major Depression and Substance Use Disorders. *Journal of Consulting and Clinical Psychology, 65,* 328–332.

Grossman, H. (1983). *Classification in Mental Retardation* (3rd rev.). Washington, DC: American Association on Mental Deficiency.

Gupta, R., & Derevensky, J. L. (1996). The relationship between gambling and video-game playing behavior in children and adolescents. *Journal of Gambling Studies, 12,* 375–394.

Guzder, J., Paris, J., Zelkowitz, P., & Marchessault, K. (1996). Risk factors for borderline pathology in children. *Journal of the American Academy of Child and Adolescent Psychiatry, 35,* 26–33.

Hall, A., Slim, E., Hawker, F., & Salmond, C. (1984). Anorexia Nervosa: Long-term outcome in 50 female patients. *British Journal of Psychiatry, 145,* 407–413.

Halperin, J. M., Matier, K., Bedi, G., Sharma, V., & Newcorn, J. H. (1992). Specificity of inattention, impulsivity, and hyperactivity to the diagnosis of Attention-Deficit Hyperactivity Disorder. *Journal of the American Academy of Child and Adolescent Psychiatry, 31,* 190–196.

Halperin, J. M., Newcorn, J. H., Sharma, V., Healey, J. M., Wolf, L. E., Pascualvaca, D. M., & Schwartz, S. (1990). Inattentive and noninattentive ADHD children: Do they constitute a unitary group? *Journal of Abnormal Child Psychology, 18,* 437–449.

Hardman, M. L., Drew, C. J., & Egan, M. W. (1996). *Human exceptionality: Society, school, and family* (5th ed.). Needham Heights, MA: Allyn & Bacon.

Harris, S. L., Glasberg, B., & Ricca, D. (1996). Pervasive Developmental Disorders: Distinguishing among subtypes. *School Psychology Review, 25,* 308–315.

Hasin, D., McCloud, S., Qun, L., & Endicott, J. (1996). Cross-system agreement among demographic subgroups: DSM-III, DSM-III-R, DSM-IV, and ICD-10 diagnoses of alcohol use disorders. *Drug and Alcohol Dependence, 41,* 127–135.

Hayward, C., Killen, J. D., Kramer, H. C., Blair-Greiner, A., Strachowski, D., Cunning, D., & Taylor, C. B. (1997). Assessment and phenomenology of nonclinical Panic Attacks in adolescent girls. *Journal of Anxiety Disorders, 11,* 17–32.

Heber, R. (1959). A manual on terminology and classification in Mental Retardation (rev.). *American Journal of Mental Deficiency, 56*(Monograph Suppl.).

Heber, R. (1961). Modifications in the manual on terminology and classification in Mental Retardation. *American Journal of Mental Deficiency, 65,* 499–500.

Hellgren, L., Gillberg, I. C., Bahenholm, A., & Gillberg, C. (1994). Children with deficits in attention, motor control and perception (DAMP) almost grown up: Psychiatric and personality disorders at age 16 years. *Journal of Child Psychiatry and Psychology, 35,* 1255–1271.

Henderson, S. E., Barnett, A., & Henderson, L. (1994). Visuospatial difficulties and clumsiness: On the interpretation of conjoined deficits. *Journal of Child Psychiatry and Psychology, 35,* 961–969.

Herbert, J. (1995). An overview of the current status of social phobia. *Applied and Preventive Psychology, 4,* 39–51.

Hinshaw, S. P. (1992). Academic underachievement, attention deficits, and aggression: Comorbidity and implications for intervention. *Journal of Consulting and Clinical Psychology, 60,* 893–903.

Hodapp, R. M. (1995). Definitions in Mental Retardation: Effects on research, practice, and perceptions. *School Psychology Quarterly, 10,* 24–28.

Hooper, S. R., & Willis, W. G. (1989). *Learning disability subtyping: Neuropsychological foundations, conceptual models, and issues in clinical differentiation.* New York: Springer-Verlag.

Horowitz, M., Siegel, B., Holen, A., Bonanno, G. A., Milbrath, C., & Stinson,

C. H. (1997). Diagnostic criteria for Complicated Grief Disorder. *American Journal of Psychiatry, 154,* 904–910.

Horwitz, S. M., Bility, K. M., Plichta, S. B., Leaf, P. J., & Haynes, N. (1998). Teacher assessments of children's behavioral disorders: Demographic correlates. *American Journal of Orthopsychiatry, 68,* 117–125.

Illinois State Board of Education. (2001). *A parents' guide: The educational rights of students with disabilities.* Springfield, IL: Special Education Compliance Division.

Isaac, G. (1991). Bipolar Disorder in prepubertal children in a special education setting: Is it rare? *Journal of Clinical Psychiatry, 52,* 165–168.

Jacobson, J. W. (1982). Problem behavior and psychiatric impairment in a developmentally disabled population: I. Behavior frequency. *Applied Research in Mental Retardation, 3,* 121–139.

Jensen, P. S., & Hoagwood, K. (1997). The book of names: DSM-IV in context. *Development and Psychopathology, 9,* 231–249.

Jordan, F. M., Murdoch, B. E., Buttsworth, D. L., & Hudson-Tennent, L. J. (1995). Speech and language performance of brain-injured children. *Aphasiology, 9,* 23–32.

Jordan, F. M., Ozanne, A. E., & Murdoch, B. E. (1988). Long term speech and language disorders subsequent to closed head injury in children. *Brain Injury, 2,* 179–185.

Jordan, F. M., Ozanne, A. E., & Murdoch, B. E. (1990). Performance of closed head–injured children on a naming task. *Brain Injury, 4,* 27–32.

Kashani, J. H., Allan, W. D., Beck, N. C. Jr., Bledsoe, Y., & Reid, J. C. (1997). Dysthymic Disorder in clinically referred preschool children. *Journal of the American Academy of Child and Adolescent Psychiatry, 36,* 1426–1433.

Kashani, J. H., Holcomb, W. R., & Orvaschel, H. (1986). Depression and depressive symptoms in preschool children from the general population. *American Journal of Psychiatry, 143,* 1138–1143.

Katon, W. (1993). Somatization Disorder, Hypochondriasis, and Conversion Disorder. In D. Dunner (Ed.), *Current psychiatric therapy.* Philadelphia: Saunders.

Kay, S. R. (1989). Cognitive battery for differential diagnosis of Mental Retardation vs. psychosis. *Research in Developmental Disabilities, 10,* 251–260.

Kearney, C., Albano, A. M., Eisen, A. R., Allan, W. D., & Barlow, D. H. (1997). The phenomenology of Panic Disorder in youngsters: An empirical study of a clinical sample. *Journal of Anxiety Disorders, 11,* 49–62.

Keller, M. B. (1994). Course, outcome and impact on the community. *Acta Psychiatrica Scandinavica, 89,* 24–34.

Kerwin, M. E., & Berkowitz, R. I. (1996). Feeding and eating disorders: Ingestive problems of infancy, childhood, and adolescence. *School Psychology Review, 25,* 316–328.

Khan, A., Cowan, C., & Roy, A. (1997). Personality Disorders in people with learning disabilities: A community survey. *Journal of Intellectual Disability Research, 41,* 324–330.

King, B. H., DeAntonio, C., McCracken, J. T., Forness, S. R., & Ackerland, V. (1994). Psychiatric consultation in Severe and Profound Mental Retardation. *American Journal of Psychiatry, 151,* 1802–1808.

King, B. H., State, M. W., Shah, B., Davanzo, P., & Dykens, E., (1997). Mental Retardation: A review of the past 10 years. Part I. *Journal of the American Academy of Child and Adolesent Psychiatry, 36,* 1656–1663.

King, R. A., Scahill, L., Vitulano, L. A., Schwab-Stone, M., Tercyak, K. P., & Riddle, M. A. (1995). Childhood Trichotillomania: Clinical phenomenology, comorbidity, and family genetics. *Journal of the American Academy of Child and Adolesent Psychiatry, 34,* 1451–1459.

Kirk, S. A. & Kutchins, H. (1992). *The selling of DSM: The rhetoric of science in psychiatry.* New York: Aldine de Gruyter.

Klin, A., Volkmar, F. R., Sparrow, S. S., Cicchetti, D. V., & Rourke, B. P. (1995). Validity and neuropsychological characterization of Asperger syndrome: Convergence with nonverbal learning disabilities syndrome. *Journal of Child Psychiatry and Psychology, 36,* 1127–1140.

Kluft, R. P. (1984). Multiple Personality in childhood. *Psychiatric Clinics of North America, 7*(1), 121–134.

Knights, R. M., Ivan, L. P., Ventureyra, E. C. G., Bentivoglio, C., Stoddart, C., Winogron, W., & Bawden, H. N. (1991). The effects of head injury in children on neuropsychological and behavioral functioning. *Brain Injury, 5,* 339–351.

Koerner, K., Kohlenberg, R. J., & Parker, C. R. (1996). Diagnosis of Personality Disorder: A radical behavioral alternative. *Journal of Consulting and Clinical Psychology, 64,* 1169–1176.

Kopp, S., & Gillberg, C. (1997). Selective Mutism: A population-based study: A research note. *Journal of Child Psychology and Psychiatry, 38,* 257–262.

Kraus, J. F., Fife, D., & Conroy, C. (1987). Pediatric brain injuries: The nature, clinical course, and early outcomes in a defined United States population. *Pediatrics, 79,* 501–507.

Kraus, J. F., Rock, A., & Hemyari, P. (1990). Brain injuries among infants, children, adolescents, and young adults. *American Journal of Diseases of Children, 144,* 684–691.

Kronenberger, W. G., & Meyer, R. G. (1996). *The child clinician's handbook.* Needham Heights, MA: Allyn & Bacon.

Kutchins, H., & Kirk, S. A. (1995). DSM-IV: Does bigger and newer mean better? *Harvard Mental Health Letter, 11,* 4–6.

Lahey, B. B., Applegate, B., McBurnett, K, Biederman, J., Greenhill, L., Hynd, G. W., Barkley, R. A., Newcorn, J., Jensen, P., Richters, J., Garfinkel, B., Kerdyk, L., Frick, P. J., Ollendick, T., Perez, D., Hart, E. L., Waldman, I., & Shaffer, D. (1994). DSM-IV field trials for Attention-Deficit/Hyperactivity Disorder in children and adolescents. *American Journal of Psychiatry, 151,* 1673–1685.

Lahey, B. B., Loeber, R., Quay, H. C., Frick, P. J., & Grimm, J. (1992). Oppositional-Defiant and Conduct Disorders: Issues to be resolved in DSM-IV. *Journal of the American Academy of Child and Adolescent Psychiatry, 31,* 539–545.

Lahey, B. B., Schaughency, E., Hynd, G., Carlson, C., & Nieves, N. (1987). Attention Deficit Disorder with and without Fyperactivity: Comparison of behavioral characteristics of clinic–referred children. *Journal of the American Academy of Child Psychiatry, 26,* 718–723.

Lahey, B. B., Schaughency, E., Strauss, C., & Frame, C. L. (1984). Are Attention Deficit Disorders with and without Hyperactivity similar or dissimilar? *Journal of the American Academy of Child Psychiatry, 23,* 302–309.

Langer, L.M., & Tubman, J. G. (1997). Risky sexual behavior among substance-abusing adolescents: Psychosocial and contextual factors. *American Journal of Orthopsychiatry, 67,* 315–322.

Last, C. G., Francis, G., Hersen, M., Kazdin, A. E., & Strauss, C. C. (1987). Separation anxiety and school phobia: A comparison using DSM-III criteria. *American Journal of Psychiatry, 144,* 653–657.

Leeper, L. H. (1992). Diagnostic examination of children with voice disorders: A low-cost solution. *Language, Speech, and Hearing Services in Schools, 23,* 353–360.

Lehmkuhl, G., Blanz, B., Lehmkuhl, U., & Braum–Scharm, H. (1989). Conversion Disorder (DSM-III 300.11): Symptomatology and course in childhood and adolescence. *European Archives of Psychiatry and Neurological Sciences, 238,* 155–160.

Levy, F., Hay, D. A., McStephen, M., Wood, C., & Waldman, I. (1997). Attention-Deficit Hyperactivity Disorder: A category or a continuum? Genetic analysis of a large-scale twin study. *Journal of the American Academy of Child and Adolescent Psychiatry, 36,* 737–744.

Lewinsohn, P. M., Rohde, P., & Seeley, J. R. (1995). Adolescent psychopathology: III. The clinical consequences of comorbidity. *Journal of the American Academy of Child and Adolescent Psychiatry, 34,* 510–519.

Lewinsohn, P. M., Rohde, P., Seeley, J. R., & Klein, D. N. (1997). Axis II psychopathology as a function of Axis I disorders in childhood and adolescence. *Journal of the American Academy of Child and Adolescent Psychiatry, 36,* 1752–1759.

Lewis, M. (1996). Borderline features in childhood disorders. In F. R. Volkmar (Ed.), *Psychoses and Pervasive Developmental Disorders in childhood and adolescence.* Washington, DC: American Psychiatric Press.

Lewis, D. O., Lewis, M., Unger, L., & Goldman, C. (1984). Conduct Disorder and its synonyms: Diagnoses of dubious validity and usefulness. *American Journal of Psychiatry, 141,* 514–519.

Linehan, M. M. (1993). *Cognitive-behavioral treatment of Borderline Personality Disorder.* New York: Guilford Press.

Loeber, R., Lahey, B. B., & Thomas, C. (1991). Diagnostic conundrum of Oppositional-Defiant Disorder and Conduct Disorder. *Journal of Abnormal Psychology, 100,* 379–390.

Ludolph, P. S., Westen, D., Misle, B., Jackson, A., Wixom, J., & Wiss, F. C. (1990). The borderline diagnosis in adolescents: Symptoms and developmental history. *American Journal of Psychiatry, 147,* 470–476.

Lynam, D. R. (1996). Early identification of the chronic offender: Who is the fledgling psychopath? *Psychological Bulletin, 120,* 209–234.

Lynskey, M., & Fergusson, D. M. (1995). Childhood conduct problems, attention deficit behaviors, and adolescent alcohol, tobacco, and illicit drug use. *Journal of Abnormal Child Psychology, 23,* 281–302.

MacMillan, D. L., Gresham, F. M., & Siperstein, G. N. (1993). Conceptual and psychometric concerns about the 1992 AAMR definition of Mental Retardation. *American Journal of Mental Retardation, 98*, 325–335.

MacMillan, D. L., Gresham, F. M., Siperstein, G. N., & Bocian, K. M. (1996). The labyrinth of IDEA: School decisions on referred students with subaverage general intelligence. *American Journal of Mental Retardation, 101*, 161–174.

March, J. S. (1993). What constitutes a stressor? The "Criterion A" issue. In J. R. T. Davidson & E. B. Foa (Eds.), *Posttraumatic Stress Disorder: DSM–IV and beyond.* Washington, DC: American Psychiatric Press.

March, J. S., & Leonard, H. L. (1996). Obsessive–Compulsive Disorder in children and adolescents: A review of the past 10 years. *Journal of the American Academy of Child and Adolescent Psychiatry, 35*, 1265–1273.

Marks, I. (1988). Blood–injury phobia: A review. *American Journal of Psychiatry, 145*, 1207–1213.

Matson, J. L. (1995). Comments on Gresham, MacMillan, and Siperstein's paper "Critical analysis of the 1992 AAMR definition: Implications for school psychology." *School Psychology Quarterly, 10*, 20–23.

Max, J. E., & Dunisch, D. L. (1997). Traumatic brain injury in a child psychiatry outpatient clinic: A controlled study. *Journal of the American Academy of Child and Adolescent Psychiatry, 36*, 404–411.

Max, J. E., Robin, D. A., Lindgren, S. D., Smith, W. L., Sato, Y., Mattheis, P. J., Stierwalt, J. A. G., & Castillo, C. S. (1997). Traumatic brain injury in children and adolescents: Psychiatric disorders at two years. *Journal of the American Academy of Child and Adolescent Psychiatry, 36*, 1278–1285.

Max, J. E., Sharma, A., & Qurashi, M. I. (1997). Traumatic brain injury in a child psychiatric inpatient population: A controlled study. *Journal of the American Academy of Child and Adolescent Psychiatry, 36*, 1595–1601.

Max, J. E., Smith, W. L., Sato, Y., Mattheis, P. J., Castillo, C. S., Lindgren, S. D., Robin, D. A., & Stierwalt, J. A. G. (1997). Traumatic brain injury in children and adolescents: Psychiatric disorders in the first three months. *Journal of the American Academy of Child and Adolescent Psychiatry, 36*, 94–102.

McBurnett, K., Lahey, B. B., & Pfiffner, L. J. (1993). Diagnosis of attention deficit disorders in DSM-IV: Scientific basis and implications for education. *Exceptional Children, 60*, 108–117.

McGarvey, E. L., Canterbury, R. J., & Waite, D. (1996). Delinquency and family problems in incarcerated adolescents with and without a history of inhalant use. *Addictive Behavior, 21*, 537–542.

McGinnis, E. (1986). *The relationship between psychiatric hospitalization and special education placement.* Unpublished doctoral dissertation, University of Iowa.

McGlashan, T. H. (1988). Adolescent versus adult onset of mania. *American Journal of Psychiatry, 145*, 221–223.

McGrath, P. M. (1995). Annotation: Aspects of pain in children and adolescents. *Journal of Child Psychiatry and Psychology, 36*, 717–730.

McNally, R. J. (1993). Stressors that produce Posttraumatic Stress Disorder in children. In J. R. T. Davidson & E. B. Foa (Eds.), *Posttraumatic*

Stress Disorder: DSM-IV and beyond. Washington, DC: American Psychiatric Press.

Menolascino, F. J. (1988). Mental illness in the mentally retarded: Diagnostic and treatment issues. In J. A. Stark, F. J. Menolascino, M. H. Albarelli, & V. C. Gray (Eds.), *Mental Retardation and mental health: Classification, diagnosis, treatment, services.* New York: Springer-Verlag.

Meyer, R. G,. & Deitsch, S. E. (1996). *The clinician's handbook: Integrated diagnostics, assessment, and intervention in adult and adolescent psychopathology* (4th ed.). Needham Heights, MA: Allyn & Bacon.

Miller, L. C., Barrett, C. L., & Hampe, E. (1974). Phobias of childhood in a prescientific era. In A. Davids (Ed.), *Child personality and psychopathology: Current topics* (Vol. 1). New York: Wiley.

Milne, J. M., Garrison, C. Z., Addy, C. L., McKeown, R. E., Jackson, K. L., Cuffe, S. P., & Waller, J. L. (1995). Frequency of phobic disorder in a community sample of young adolescents. *Journal of the American Academy of Child and Adolescent Psychiatry, 34,* 1202–1211.

Mischel, W. (1968). *Personality and assessment.* New York: Wiley.

Morgan, S. B. (1990). Early childhood autism: Current perspectives on definition, assessment, and treatment. In S. B. Morgan & T. M. Okwumabua (Eds.), *Child and adolescent disorders: Developmental and health psychology perspectives.* Hillsdale, NJ: Erlbaum.

Motta, R. W. (1995). Childhood Posttraumatic Stress Disorder and the schools. *Canadian Journal of School Psychology, 11,* 65–78.

Mrazek, D. A. (1994). Psychiatric aspects of somatic disease and disorders. In M. Rutter, E. Taylor, & L. Hersov (Eds.), *Child and adolescent psychiatry: Modern approaches.* Oxford: Blackwell.

Myklebust, H. R. (1975). Nonverbal learning disabilities: Assessment and intervention. In H. R. Myklebust (Ed.), *Progress in learning disabilities* (Vol. 3). New York: Grune & Stratton.

Newcomb, M. D., & Bentler, P. M. (1989). Substance use and abuse among children and teenagers. *American Psychologist, 44,* 242–248.

Newcorn, J. H., & Strain, J. (1992). Adjustment Disorder in children and adolescents. *Journal of the American Academy of Child and Adolescent Psychiatry, 31,* 318–327.

Nordyke, N. S., Baer, D. M., Etzel, B. C., & LeBlanc, J. M. (1977). Implications of the stereotyping of modification of sex role. *Journal of Applied Behavior Analysis, 10,* 553–557.

Novins, D. K., Bechtold, D. W., Sack, W. H., Thompson, J., Carter, D. R., & Manson, S. M. (1997). The DSM-IV outline for cultural formulation: A critical demonstration with American Indian children. *Journal of the American Academy of Child and Adolescent Psychiatry, 36,* 1244–1251.

Nurcombe, B., Mitchell, W., Begtrup, R., Tramontana, M., LaBarbera, J., & Pruitt, J. (1996). Dissociative Hallucinosis and allied conditions. In F. R. Volkmar (Ed.), *Psychoses and Pervasive Developmental Disorders in childhood and adolescence.* Washington, DC: American Psychiatric Press.

Oakland, T. (1992). School dropouts: Characteristics and prevention. *Applied and Preventive Psychology, 1,* 201–208.

Othmer, E., & Othmer, S. C. (1994a). *The clinical interview using DSM–IV: Vol. 1. Fundamentals.* Washington, DC: American Psychiatric Press.

Othmer, E., & Othmer, S. C. (1994b). *The clinical interview using DSM–IV: Vol. 2. The difficult patient.* Washington, DC: American Psychiatric Press.

Palla, B., & Litt, I. R. (1988). Medical complications of Eating Disorders in adolescents. *Pediatrics, 81,* 613–623.

Paul, R. (1995). *Language disorders: From infancy through adolescence.* St. Louis, MO: Mosby.

Pauls, D. L., Alsobrook, J. P., II, Goodman, W., Rasmussen, S., & Leckman, J. F. (1995). A family study of Obsessive–Compulsive Disorder. *American Journal of Psychiatry, 152,* 76–84.

Pavkov, T. W., Lewis, D. A., & Lyons, J. S. (1989). Psychiatric diagnosis and racial bias: An empirical investigation. *Professional Psychology: Research and Practice, 20,* 364–368.

Pfeffer, C. R. (1992). Relationship between depression and suicidal behavior. In M. Shafii & S. L. Shafii (Eds.), *Clinical guide to depression in children and adolescents.* Washington, DC: American Psychiatric Press.

Pfefferbaum, B. (1997). Posttraumatic Stress Disorder in children: A review of the past 10 years. *Journal of the American Academy of Child and Adolescent Psychiatry, 36,* 1503–1511.

Pietrini, P., Dani, A., Furey, M. L., Alexander, G. E., Freo, U., Grady, C. L., Mentis, M. J., Mangot, D., Simon, E. W., Horwitz, B., Haxby, J. V., & Schapiro, M. B. (1997). Low glucose metabolism during brain stimulation in older Down's syndrome subjects at risk for Alzheimer's disease prior to dementia. *American Journal of Psychiatry, 154,* 1063–1069.

Pilowsky, D. (1986). Problems in determining the presence of hallucinations in children. In D. Pilowsky & W. Chambers (Eds.), *Hallucinations in children.* Washington, DC: American Psychiatric Press.

Power, T. J., & DuPaul, G. J. (1996a). Implications of DSM-IV for the practice of school psychology: Introduction to the mini-series. *School Psychology Review, 25,* 255–258.

Power, T. J., & DuPaul, G. J. (1996b). Attention-Deficit Hyperactivity Disorder: The reemergence of subtypes. *School Psychology Review, 25,* 284–296.

Putnam, F. W. (1996). Posttraumatic Stress Disorder in children and adolescents. In L. J. Dickstein, M. B. Riba, & J. M. Oldham (Eds.), *Review of psychiatry* (Vol. 15). Washington, DC: American Psychiatric Press.

Putnam, F. W., Helmers, K., & Trickett, P. K. (1993). Development, reliability and validity of a child dissociation scale. *Child Abuse and Neglect, 17,* 731–741.

Rapoport, J. L. (1997). What is known about childhood Schizophrenia? *Harvard Mental Health Letter, 14,* 8.

Reeves, R. R., & Bullen, J. A. (1995). Mnemonics for ten DSM-IV disorders. *Journal of Nervous and Mental Disease, 183,* 550–551.

Reid, R. (1995). Assessment of ADHD with culturally different groups: The use of behavioral rating scales. *School Psychology Review, 24,* 537–560.

Reiss, S. (1994a). Issues in defining Mental Retardation. *American Journal on Mental Retardation, 99,* 1–7.

Reiss, S. (1994b). Psychopathology in Mental Retardation. In N. Bouras (Ed.), *Mental health in Mental Retardation: Recent advances and practices.* Cambridge, England: Cambridge University Press.

Rekers, G. A., & Lovaas, I. O. (1974). Behavioral treatment of deviant sex role behaviors in a male child. *Journal of Applied Behavior Analysis, 7,* 173–190.

Rivara, J. B., Jaffe, K. M., Fay, G. C., Polissar, N. L., Martin, K. M., Shurtleff, H. A., & Liao, S. (1993). Family functioning and injury severity as predictors of child functioning one year following traumatic brain injury. *Archives of Physical Medicine and Rehabilitation, 74,* 1047–1055.

Roberts, M. A. (1990). A behavioral observation method for differentiating hyperactive and aggressive boys. *Journal of Abnormal Child Psychology, 18,* 131–142.

Robins, L. R. (1991). Conduct disorder. *Journal of Child Psychiatry and Psychology, 32,* 1193–212.

Rourke, B. P. (1987). Syndrome of nonverbal learning disabilities: The final common pathway of white-matter disease/dysfunction? *The Clinical Neuropsychologist, 1,* 209–234.

Rourke, B. P. (1988). The syndrome of nonverbal learning disabilities: Developmental manifestations in neurological disease, disorder, and dysfunction. *The Clinical Neuropsychologist, 2,* 293–330.

Rourke, B. P. (1989). *Nonverbal learning disabilities: The syndrome and the model.* New York: Guilford Press.

Rourke, B. P., Del Dotto, J. E., Rourke, S. B., & Casey, J. E. (1990). Nonverbal learning disabilities: The syndrome and a case study. *Journal of School Psychology, 28,* 361–385.

Russell, A. T., Bott, L., & Sammons, C. (1989). The phenomenology of Schizophrenia occurring in childhood. *Journal of the American Academy of Child and Adolescent Psychiatry, 28,* 399–407.

Rutter, M. (1981). Psychological sequelae of brain damage in children. *American Journal of Psychiatry, 138,* 1533–1544.

Ryan, N. D., Puig-Antich, J., Ambrosini, P., Rabinovich, H., Robinson, D., Nelson, B., Iyengar, S., & Twomey, J. (1987). The clinical picture of Major Depression in children and adolescents. *Archives of General Psychiatry, 44,* 854–861.

Sabatino, D. A., & Vance, H. B. (1994). Is the diagnosis of Attention-Deficit/Hyperactivity Disorder meaningful? *Psychology in the Schools, 31,* 188–196.

Sands, R., Tricker, J., Sherman, C., Armatas, C., & Maschette, W. (1997). Disordered eating patterns, body image, self-esteem, and physical activity in preadolescent school children. *International Journal of Eating Disorders, 21,* 159–166.

Sarma, P. S. B. (1994). Physical and neurological examinations and laboratory studies. In K. S. Robson (Ed.), *Manual of clinical child and adolescent psychiatry* (rev. ed.). Washington, DC: Amerian Psychiatric Press.

Scheeringa, M. S., Zeanah, C. H., Drell, M. J., & Larrieu, J. A. (1995). Two approaches to the diagnosis of Posttraumatic Stress Disorder in infancy and early childhood. *Journal of the American Academy of Child and Adolescent Psychiatry, 34,* 191–200.

Schmidt, C. W., Jr. (1993). *CPT handbook for psychiatrists.* Washington, DC: American Psychiatric Press.

Schwarz, E. D., & Kowalski, J. M. (1991). Posttraumatic Stress Disorder after a school shooting: Effects of symptom threshold selection and diagnosis by DSM-III, DSM-III-R, or proposed DSM-IV. *American Journal of Psychiatry, 148,* 592–597.

Scott, S. (1994). Mental Retardation. In M. Rutter, E. Taylor, & L. Hersov (Eds.), *Child and adolescent psychiatry: Modern approaches.* Oxford: Blackwell.

Scotti, J. R., Morris, T. L., McNeil, C. B., & Hawkins, R. P. (1996). DSM-IV and disorders of childhood and adolescence: Can structural criteria be functional? *Journal of Consulting and Clinical Psychology, 64,* 1177–1191.

Semrud-Klikeman, M., & Hynd, G. W. (1990). Right hemispheric dysfunction in nonverbal learning disabilities: Social, academic, and adaptive functioning in adults and children. *Psychological Bulletin, 107,* 196–209.

Shaffer, H. J., LaBrie, R., Scanlan, K. M., & Cummings, T. N. (1994). Pathological gambling among adolescents: Massachusetts Gambling Screen (MAGS). *Journal of Gambling Studies, 10,* 339–362.

Shamsie, J., & Hluchy, C. (1991). Youth with Conduct Disorder: A challenge to be met. *Canadian Journal of Psychiatry, 36,* 405–414.

Shaywitz, S. E., Escobar, M. E., Shaywitz, B. A., Fletcher, J. M., & Makuch, R. (1990). Evidence that dyslexia may represent the lower tail of a normal distribution of reading ability. *New England Journal of Medicine, 326,* 145–150.

Shaywitz, S. E., Shaywitz, B. A., Fletcher, J. M., & Escobar, M. E. (1990). Prevalence of reading disability in boys and girls: Results of the Connecticut longitudinal study. *Journal of the American Medical Association, 264,* 998–1002.

Siegel, M., & Barthel, R. P. (1986). Conversion Disorders on a child psychiatry consultation service. *Psychosomatics, 27,* 201–204.

Simeon, J. G. (1989). Depressive Disorders in children and adolescents. *Psychiatry Journal of the University of Ottawa, 14,* 356–361.

Skodol, A. E. (1989). *Problems in Differential Diagnosis: From DSM-III to DSM-III-R in clinical practice.* Washington, DC: American Psychiatric Press.

Slater, E. J., & Bassett, S. S. (1988). Adolescents with closed head injuries: A report of initial cognitive deficits. *American Journal of Diseases of Children, 142,* 1048–1051.

Small, R. F. (1993). *Maximizing third-party reimbursement in your mental health practice.* Sarasota, FL: Professional Resource Exchange.

Smart, D., Sanson, A., & Prior, M. (1996). Connections between reading disability and behavior problems: Testing temporal and casual hypotheses. *Journal of Abnormal Child Psychology, 24,* 363–383.

Spitzer, R. L., Gibbon, M., Skodol, A. E., Williams, J. B. W., & First, M. B. (1994). *DSM-IV casebook: A learning companion to the Diagnostic and statis-*

tical manual of mental disorders, fourth edition. Washington, DC: American Psychiatric Press.

Spirito, A., Brown, L., Overholser, J., & Fritz, G. (1989). Attempted suicide in adolescence: A review and critique of the literature. *Clinical Psychology Review, 9,* 335–363.

State, M. W., King, B. H., & Dykens, E. (1997). Mental Retardation: A review of the past 10 years. Part II. *Journal of the American Academy of Child and Adolescent Psychiatry, 36,* 1664–1671.

Stein, D. J. (1993). Cross-cultural psychiatry and the DSM-IV. *Comprehensive Psychiatry, 34,* 322–329.

Steiner, H., & Lock, J. (1998). Anorexia nervosa and bulimia in children and adolescents: A review of the past 10 years. *Journal of the American Academy of Child and Adolescent Psychiatry, 37,* 352–359.

Steinhausen, H.-C., & Juzi, C. (1996). Elective Mutism: An analysis of 100 cases. *Journal of the American Academy of Child and Adolescent Psychiatry, 35,* 606–614.

Strauss, C. C., Lease, C. A., Last, C. G., & Francis, G. (1988). Overanxious Disorder: An examination of developmental differences. *Journal of Abnormal Child Psychology, 16,* 433–443.

Strub, R. L., & Black, F. W. (1988). *Neurobehavioral disorders: A clinical approach.* Philadelphia: F. A. Davis.

Substance Abuse and Mental Health Services Administration. (1993). Action: Final notice. *Federal Register, 58,* 29422–29425.

Swedo, S. E., Leonard, H. L., Mittleman, B. B., Allen, A. J., Rapoport, J. L., Dow, S. P., Kanter, M. E., Chapman, F., & Zabriskie, J. (1997). Identification of children with pediatric autoimmune neuropsychiatric disorders associated with streptococcal infections by a marker associated with rheumatic fever. *American Journal of Psychiatry, 154,* 110–112.

Swedo, S. E., Rapoport, J. L., Leonard, H., Lenane, M., & Cheslow, D. (1989). Obsessive–compulsive Disorder in children and adolescents: Clinical phenomenology of 70 consecutive cases. *Archives of General Psychiatry, 46,* 335–341.

Szatmari, P. (1996). Asperger's Disorder and atypical Pervasive Developmental Disorder. In F. R. Volkmar (Ed.), *Psychoses and Pervasive Developmental Disorders in childhood and adolescence.* Washington, DC: American Psychiatric Press.

Szymanski, L. S. (1994). Mental Retardation and mental health: Concepts, aetiology and incidence. In N. Bouras (Ed.), *Mental health in Mental Retardation: Recent advances and practices.* Cambridge, England: Cambridge University Press.

Thornton, C., & Russell, J. (1997). Obsessive compulsive comorbidity in the dieting disorders. *International Journal of Eating Disorders, 21,* 83–87.

Tumuluru, R., Yaylayan, S., Weller, E. B., & Weller, R. A. (1996a). Affective psychoses: I. Major Depression with psychosis. In F. R. Volkmar (Ed.), *Psychoses and Pervasive Developmental Disorders in childhood and adolescence.* Washington, DC: American Psychiatric Press.

Tumuluru, R., Yaylayan, S., Weller, E. B., & Weller, R. A. (1996b). Affective psychoses: II. Bipolar Disorder with psychosis. In F. R. Volkmar (Ed.), *Psychoses and Pervasive Developmental Disorders in childhood and adolescence.* Washington, DC: American Psychiatric Press.

Turkat, I. D. (1990). *The Personality Disorders: A psychological approach to clinical management.* New York: Pergamon Press.

Turner, R. P., Lukoff, D., Barnhouse, R. T., & Lu, F. G. (1995). Religious or Spiritual Problem: A culturally sensitive diagnostic category in the DSM-IV. *Journal of Nervous and Mental Diseases, 183,* 435–444.

U.S. Department of Education. (1991). Notice of proposed rulemaking. *Federal Register, 56*(160), 41271.

U.S. Department of Health, Education and Welfare. (1977). Education of Handicapped Children (Implementation of Part B of the Education of the Handicapped Act). *Federal Register, 42*(163), 42478.

van Goor-Lambo, G. (1987). The reliability of Axis V of the multiaxial classification scheme. *Journal of Child Psychology and Psychiatry, 28,* 597–612.

Vitiello, B., & Stoff, D. M. (1997). Subtypes of aggression and their relevance to child psychiatry. *Journal of the American Academy of Child and Adolescent Psychiatry, 36,* 307–315.

Volkmar, F. R. (1996). The disintegrative disorders: Childhood Disintegrative Disorder and Rett's Disorder. In F. R. Volkmar (Ed.), *Psychoses and Pervasive Developmental Disorders in childhood and adolescence.* Washington, DC: American Psychiatric Press.

Volkmar, F. R., Bregman, J., Cohen, D. J., & Cicchetti, D. V. (1988). DSM-III and DSM-III-R diagnoses of Autism. *American Journal of Psychiatry, 145,* 1404–1408.

Volkmar, F. R., Klin, A., Marans, W. D., & McDougle, C. J. (1996). Autistic Disorder. In F. R. Volkmar (Ed.), *Psychoses and Pervasive Developmental Disorders in childhood and adolescence.* Washington, DC: American Psychiatric Press.

Volkmar, F. R., Klin, A., Schultz, R., Bronen, R., Maran, W. D., Sparrow, S., & Cohen, D. J. (1996). Asperger's syndrome. *Journal of the American Academy of child and adolescent Psychiatry, 35,* 118–123.

Volkmar, F. R., & Rutter, M. (1995). Childhood Disintegrative Disorder: Results of the DSM-IV autism field trial. *Journal of the American Academy of Child and Adolescent Psychiatry, 34,* 1092–1095.

Waldman, I. D., & Lilienfeld, S. O. (1995). Diagnosis and classification. In M. Hersen & R. T. Ammerman (Eds.), *Advanced abnormal child psychology.* Hillsdale, NJ: Erlbaum.

Walter, A. L., & Carter, A. S. (1997). Gilles de la Tourette's syndrome in childhood: A guide for school professionals. *School Psychology Review, 26,* 28–46.

Weinberg, W. A., & Brumback, R. A. (1976). Mania in childhood: Case studies and literature review. *American Journal of Diseases of Children, 130,* 380–385.

Werry, J. S. (1996). Childhood Schizophrenia. In F. R. Volkmar (Ed.), *Psychoses and Pervasive Developmental Disorders in childhood and adolescence.* Washington, DC: American Psychiatric Press.

Westen, D., Ludolph, P., Lerner, H., Ruffins, S., & Wiss, F. C. (1990). Object relations in borderline adolescents. *Journal of the American Academy of Child and Adolescent Psychiatry, 29,* 338–348.

Wiederman, M. W., & Pryor, T. (1996). Substance use and impulsive behaviors among adolescents with Eating Disorders. *Addictive Behaviors, 21,* 269–272.

Wolfe, B. E. (1979). Behavioral treatment of childhood gender disorders. *Behavior Modification, 4,* 550–575.

Wolpe, J. (1990). *The practice of behavior therapy* (4th ed.). New York: Pergamon Press.

World Health Organization. (1977). *Manual of the international statistical classification of diseases, injuries, and causes of death* (9th rev., 2 vols.). Geneva: Author.

World Health Organization. (1991). *International classification of diseases—clinical modification* (9th rev., 4th ed., 2 vols.). Washington, DC: U.S. Department of Health and Human Services.

World Health Organization. (1992a). *Manual of the international statistical classification of diseases and related health problems* (10th rev., 3 vols.). Geneva: Author.

World Health Organization. (1992b). *The ICD-10 classification of mental and behavioural disorders: Clinical descriptions and diagnostic guidelines.* Geneva: Author.

Wulfert, E., Greenway, D. E., & Dougher, M. J. (1996). A logical functional analysis of reinforcement-based disorders: Alcoholism and Pedophilia. *Journal of Consulting and Clinical Psychology, 64,* 1140–1151.

Wynick, S., Hobson, R. P., & Jones, R. B. (1997). Psychogenic disorders of vision in childhood ("visual conversion reactions"): Perspectives from adolescence. A research note. *Journal of Child Psychiatry and Psychology, 38,* 375–379.

Yorkston, K. M., Jaffe, K. M., Polissar, N. L., Liao, S., & Fay, G. C. (1997). Written language production and neuropsychological function in children with traumatic brain injury. *Archives of Physical Medicine and Rehabilitation, 78,* 1096–1102.

Young, J. E. (1990). *Cognitive therapy for Personality Disorders: A schema-focused approach.* Sarasota, FL: Professional Resources Exchange.

Zoccolillo, M., Meyers, J., & Assiter, S. (1997). Conduct disorder, substance dependence, and adolescent motherhood. *American Journal of Orthopsychiatry, 67,* 152–157.

Zucker, K. J. (1990). Treatment of Gender Identity Disorders in children. In R. Blanchard & B. W. Steiner (Eds.), *Clinical management of Gender Identity Disorders in children and adults.* Washington, DC: American Psychiatric Association.

Index

◆

2002 Updates:
IDEA 1997 and DSM-IV-TR

◆

OVERVIEW

The basic elements of IDEA 1997 are consistent with the framework of the original 1977 legislation. Most of the changes have to do with the application of the act and modifications to ensure proper provision of services. There were some changes in the definition of qualifying conditions that could be related to DSM-IV diagnoses. The most important concern children diagnosed with Attention-Deficit/Hyperactivity Disorder (ADHD) and Conduct Disorder.

The appearance of DSM-IV-TR in 2000 created a stir within the mental health community. The previous publication of a "midcycle" revision, when many of the categories of DSM-III (American Psychiatric Association, 1980) were significantly altered in DSM-III-R (American Psychiatric Association, 1987), had not been well received by a number of investigators. They argued that research based on the DSM-III categories was just beginning to reach publication, and that there was not a sufficient empirical basis for change after only 7 years. The fallout from this debate were pronouncements that there would be no DSM-IV-R.

So, what is this DSM-IV-TR? What has changed? Not, with only a few exceptions, the diagnostic categories themselves. The diagnostic criteria—the symptoms, the thresholds, the exclusions, the subtypes, and the qualifiers—are (almost) all identical to the statements in DSM-IV. The practicing clinician can continue using the diagnostic criteria of DSM-IV with confidence, or can shift to a copy of DSM-IV-TR without missing a beat. The basic change, indicated in the title revision, has been to the text of DSM-IV, not to the diagnostic criteria. The major alterations have been the updating of the text material to reflect the growth of knowledge in the field of psychopathology over the past few years. The discussions of syndromes, their associated characteristics, cultural and gender features, course, and familial pattern have all been revised to the extent that reliable new information has emerged from research in the field.

This gives the reader of DSM-IV-TR a more up-to-date view of mental health classification, but does it affect the diagnoses reached by a practitioner? Probably the answer to this question is "no" the vast majority of the time, but possibly the answer is "yes" in a few narrow ways. For instance, the "impairment or distress" criterion was removed from Tourette's Disorder. This appears to be the only change of specific diagnostic criteria in DSM-IV-TR. The change appears to have been justified, probably makes it slightly easier to honestly apply this classification where it is warranted, and likely will make very little difference in the real-world use of DSM-IV. The change in the discussion of associated symptoms, however, has at least the potential for affecting the use of secondary diagnoses. The task of the diagnostician is to account for all the clinically significant information about the case. Some of this information is used to arrive at, and justify, the primary diagnosis. What of the "leftover" symptoms? Is another diagnosis necessary or are these characteristics additional features of the primary syndrome? Changes in the discussion of associated symptoms—a matter of "text" and not "criteria"—could potentially have an effect on the number of multiple diagnoses that appear to be justified by a case presentation. My impression is that this is unlikely given the textual modifications in DSM-IV-TR, but it is an empirical question and should be examined, not just debated. The important point for readers to understand is that some important considerations may be overlooked if one concludes that, since the criteria have been left unaltered, then the fundamental application will not change. The diagnostic criteria of DSM-IV are explicitly not to be used in a rote, mechanical fashion. The appropriate use of these categorical standards demands of the examiner an understanding of the context in which the diagnoses are formulated. A part of this context is the associated features of each disorder, and some of this material was changed in DSM-IV-TR.

The clearest instance of change in diagnostic practice (and a very positive one) that will result from DSM-IV-TR is in the use of the

Global Assessment of Functioning (GAF) rating on Axis V. The discussion of making the GAF rating has been appreciably expanded and improved in DSM-IV-TR. The practicing clinician is given much better guidance in arriving at a consistent and appropriate GAF score, which should definitely improve the interrater reliability of the ratings on Axis V and improve the clinical usefulness of this measure.

DSM-IV-TR Coding Notes have been added in the pages that follow to discuss how the modifications of DSM-IV-TR affect the application of the system with children and adolescents. Some of the very meaningful changes in DSM-IV-TR are not discussed, such as the correction of DSM-IV exclusion criteria that did not allow the concurrent diagnosis of Personality Change Due to a General Medical Condition with that of Dementia, because these cases are very rarely seen in youth. Overall, however, the school psychologist and other mental health professionals need to make very few changes in their diagnostic practice to remain correct in their use of DSM-IV-TR. Appendix D (pp. 829–843) in DSM-IV-TR provides a summary of the major text modifications in the revision.

Beyond the rather minor alterations in IDEA 1997 and DSM-IV-TR is a larger phenomenon that will ultimately lead to fundamental changes in our approach to mental disorders. This quiet revolution, whose impact is just beginning to be felt, has been the accumulation of a impressive and ever-growing mass of empirical data that has used the DSM-IV system to understand, follow, and relate the emotional and behavior difficulties of youth. A great deal has been learned in just the past few years about the problems and miseries that burden children and adolescents. This understanding is beginning to give our efforts to help young people a solid foundation of reliable knowledge unlike that available ever before. This will be the real story of child psychopathology in the 21st century, and DSM-IV and the revisions that succeed it will have played a role in bringing it about.

DSM-IV-TR CODING NOTE   The GAF Rating in DSM-IV-TR

The discussion of how to make a Global Assessment of Functioning (GAF) rating in DSM-IV-TR (American Psychiatric Association, 2000, pp. 32–33) is significantly improved from the material in DSM-IV. One important clarification has to do with how different considerations are weighed. The clinician is directed to consider two aspects of the client's situation: the severity of his or her symptoms and the level of functioning. When these two components would lead to different levels of rating, it is the *lower* of the two ratings that should be recorded. This explicit decision rule should help increase agreement between independent raters as well as consistency in an individual rater's scoring over time. Also added to the discussion of the GAF rating is a four-step model to guide selection of an Axis V score, which should likewise improve reliability in the application of this element of multiaxial diagnosis.

IDEA 1997 NOTE   Disruptive Behavior Disorders and IDEA 1997

As previously discussed in the IDEA Notes on Cautions about Disruptive Behavior Disorders and IDEA (p. 44) and ADHD and IDEA (p. 54), among the most strained lines of correspondence between DSM and IDEA are those pertaining to Conduct Disorders and ADHD. Neither diagnostic category was explicitly identified as a qualification for provision of special education services under IDEA. IDEA 1997 provides a new "take" on these questions, but fundamental points of disagreement remain largely unresolved.

The symptoms of ADHD may be judged to make a child eligible for special education services under the "other health impairment" category of IDEA 1997. A DSM-IV diagnosis of ADHD does not automatically lead to a determination that the child is eligible for special education services—the "medically diagnosed physical or physiological condition" must cause "educationally related problems" (cf. Illinois State Board of Education, 2001). If it can be shown that the disability negatively affects the youth's educational performance, then he or she could be ruled eligible for services. Taken on face value, this would seem to settle things: it is difficult to imagine a child with a clinical diagnosis of ADHD who did not have consequent educational problems, this would be registered under the "other health impairment" qualifier, and services would be provided. How this will actually play out is still an open issue, influenced in part by governing units' willingness to provide services for a large group of children.

IDEA 1997 would appear to exclude children with a sole diagnosis of Conduct Disorder from qualifying for special education services under the "emotional disturbance" category. The language of IDEA 1997 suggests that "social maladjustment" is not a qualifying condition for provision of special education services. Some governing units may use this to withhold services from youth with Conduct Disorder diagnoses. If the sole manifestation of the Conduct Disorder were social maladjustment, this action could be appropriate. My own conclusion is that the impact of Conduct Disorders on a child's adjustment is so often pervasively negative, and the comorbidity of Conduct Disorders with other Mental Disorders so frequent, that many or most children with Conduct Disorder diagnoses can still be legitimately qualified for special education services under IDEA 1997.

A final consideration in this regard is that IDEA 1997 is only one of the legislative acts that govern educational units and their provision of special education services. Section 504 of the Rehabilitation Act of 1973 (Public Law 93-112) and the Americans with Disabilities Act of 1990 (ADA; Public Law 101-336) both offer protections of the rights of individuals with disabilities. As with IDEA, there is not a simple formula to translate a mental health diagnosis from DSM-IV into a disability within the meaning of Section 504 or ADA; but all of these documents focus in part on problems in human performance. A well-formulated and well-documented Mental Disorder can help in establishing a disability under these acts.

DSM-IV-TR CODING NOTE   Tic Disorders in DSM-IV-TR

Three of the changes in diagnostic criteria sets in DSM-IV-TR are the removal of the "distress or impairment" criterion from the specified Tic Disorder patterns. The criteria sets for Tourette's Disorder, Chronic Motor or Vocal Tic Disorder, and Transient Tic Disorder in DSM-IV all included as criterion C the standard statement: "The disturbance causes marked distress or significant impairment in social, occupational, or other important areas of functioning" (pp. 103, 104, 105). This element has been omitted from the respective criterion sets in DSM-IV-TR. The rationale offered for the change is that this criterion was problematic because many children seen for Tic Disorders did not show marked distress or impairment. While this has been my experience as well, the deletion raises other issues. The general criteria for a Mental Disorder in DSM refer to significant impairments in adjustment or significant personal distress or a number of very specific negative outcomes that do not apply to Tic Disorders (DSM-IV, pp. xxi–xxii ; DSM-IV-TR, p. xxxi). The frank removal of these criteria from the Tic Disorders categories leads one to ask: On what basis are these behaviors conceptualized as Mental Disorders? The problem in part stems from the nature of Tic Disorders—this phenomenon lies on the boundary between psychiatry and neurology. Many readers will agree with the authors of DSM-IV-TR that the Tic Disorders can be reasonably classified as Mental Disorders, but a clearer formulation of this assignment would be useful.

DSM-IV-TR CODING NOTE   Stereotypic Movement Disorder in DSM-IV-TR

The example of "picking at skin or bodily orifices" was removed from the list of examples of a Stereotypic Movement Disorder in the text of DSM-IV-TR (p. 131). Readers are instructed to classify this behavior as an Impulse Control Disorder Not Otherwise Specified (see p. 832). Unfortunately, the example of "picking at skin or bodily orifices" was left in the diagnostic criteria set for Stereotypic Movement Disorder on p. 134. The example of "skin picking" was also added to the discussion of Impulse Control Disorder NOS on p. 677 of DSM-IV-TR. This potential confusion appears to be simply a matter of missing the deletion planned for p. 134. Despite the oversight, the intention of the authors of DSM-IV-TR appears clear.

DSM-IV-TR CODING NOTE   Sexual Disorders in DSM-IV-TR

The clinical significance criteria for several of the Paraphilias were modified in DSM-IV-TR such that acting upon these atypical sexual urges is taken as satisfying the "general impairment" criterion to establish a Mental Disorder. The behavior patterns for Pedophilia, Voyeurism, Exhibitionism, and Frotteurism are classified as a Mental Disorder either because of causing significant personal disorder or because of being acted upon. For Sexual Sadism, acting upon these urges with a nonconsenting partner, or being distressed by the urges, satisfies the clinical significance criteria. Cases of sexual Paraphilias, while certainly not common among adolescents, do come to clinical attention, and these modifications of the criterion sets appear well justified in terms of the risks associated with acting out on these impulses in our society.

DSM-IV-TR CODING NOTE Pervasive Developmental Disorder NOS in DSM-IV-TR

Modifications of text material are especially meaningful in regard to the Not Otherwise Specified diagnoses because there are no specific diagnostic criteria for these categories—the text and the essential features of the general syndrome guide the diagnosis. The discussion of Pervasive Developmental Disorder Not Otherwise Specified was altered to eliminate the possible diagnosis of a child who showed impairment in only one of the three core problem areas: reciprocal social interaction, communication skills, and stereotyped behavior patterns. This is an illustration of "language housekeeping" to clarify a possible source of confusion. The essential view of what constitutes a Pervasive Developmental Disorder remains the same.
